Everyday English for Nursing on DVD

DVDで学ぶ看護英語

Yasuko Onjohji

John Skelton

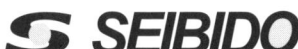

cover pictures by　表紙写真
Catherine Yeule

illustrations by　挿絵
Ruben Frosali　ルーベン・フロサリ
Takahide Joh　城 隆英

StreamLine

Web 動画・音声ファイルのストリーミング再生について

CD マーク及び Web 動画マークがある箇所は、PC、スマートフォン、タブレット端末において、無料でストリーミング再生することができます。下記 URL よりご利用ください。再生手順や動作環境などは本書巻末の「Web 動画のご案内」をご覧ください。

http://st.seibido.co.jp

音声ファイルのダウンロードについて

CD マークがある箇所は、ダウンロードすることも可能です。下記 URL より書籍を検索し、書籍詳細ページにあるダウンロードアイコンをクリックしてください。

https://www.seibido.co.jp

Movie clips and images provided
by OCBMedia, Leicester, U.K.,
in coordination with Fortuna, Inc., Japan
©OCBMedia 2009

Everyday English for Nursing on DVD

Copyright © 2009 by Yasuko Onjohji, John Skelton

*All rights reserved for Japan.
No part of this book may be reproduced in any form
without permission from Seibido Co., Ltd.*

推薦のことば

　本書は、聖路加看護大学で多年英語を教えられた園城寺康子先生とイギリスのバーミンガム大学の教職スタッフの合同作品で、看護の現場を示す動画を使用した英会話学習用のテキストです。

　患者が病院に入院してから、診察、検査の後に診断が決定して治療が行われ、リハビリテーションがなされる全行程にわたって、ナースや他の医療従事者がどのような単語を用いて会話をすれば良いケアが提供できるかの練習用テキストです。患者への挨拶やいろいろな質問をしながら、その対応の会話が示されています。耳からの上手な聞き方、患者の心身状態のとらえ方が、患者への配慮ある言葉遣いと優しい表情と共にできるようになれるか。それにはこの映像を用いることで、きわめて能率的な効果が挙げられるでしょう。

　今までにない教材として案出されたこの作品を私は絶賛します。

聖路加看護大学名誉学長
日野原重明

はじめに

　本書は看護大学や専門学校の学生を対象とした、一般的な臨床の場での会話を中心とした初級から中級レベルの教材です。看護の臨床の場での自然なコミュニケーションに焦点をしぼり、その実践を手助けすることを目指して作成したものです。欧米の看護の現場では'tacit'という言葉に象徴される暗黙のコミュニケーションを尊重する傾向もありましたが、今日では救急医療の発達やグローバル化の進展で、複雑な展開をみせ、コミュニケーションについての見方も変化してきています。イギリスでもすでに医療現場での会話の専門的分析研究が始まっており、その知見を少しでも多く活用できるように動画は編成されています。

　映像という利点を生かし、従来のオーセンティックな語学教材では学びにくい、行動、感情などを含んだ総合的コミュニケーションを、基本的な練習課題を繰り返す過程で習得できるように構成しました。特に具体的な医療場面での患者さんとの会話を、Interactive Skills という観点から捉え、リスニング力の強化も目的としています。そのため、ここではまず日常の看護での基本的な会話表現を映像でじっくり'見て覚え'、次に、内容把握、会話の呼吸、速度、音調などに注意して出来るだけ自然に会話ができるように段階的に構成しました。学習者はいつでも動画を見ることができ事前学習の課題にできる可能性も高いので、時間とレベルに応じて、新しい授業方法を開発して利用していただければ幸いです。

　この企画の発端は、イギリスのバーミンガム大学の医療コミュニケーションの専門家 John Skelton 教授の日本における講演です。その後、こちらからもバーミンガム大学の病院を訪れ、看護師の方や先生にインタビューする機会を得るという交流があり、その過程から本書が生まれました。そこにはフォルトゥーナ（株）からの提案があり、イギリスのレスター大学の協力が加わり、最終的には成美堂の佐野英一郎社長と編集の佐藤公雄氏、フォルトゥーナの高井悦夫氏のご尽力で動画付きテキストという形になりました。こちらからは場面設定と基本的会話表現を含むことを条件に設定し、実際によい会話、悪い会話、そして難しい (challenging) 場面での会話を関係者の間で行ってもらいました。その意味では、リアルなものです。スクリプト起こしと英文校閲は成美堂の Bill Benfield 氏にお願いしました。また、イギリスでの調整及び映像や音声処理はレスター大学のスタッフによるものです。

　5年間もの長きにわたり、ご協力、ご支援をして下さったこれら多くのイギリスと日本の関係者の皆様に心から感謝申し上げます。

著　者

本書の構成と使い方

I Key Sentences

各ユニットの warming-up には使用頻度の高い重要な文章をとりだしました。動画のリスニングでも聞き取れるように、その意味を確認して声に出して読み、しっかり覚えて欲しいと思います。

II Improve Your Communication Skills

この部分はイギリスで作成したこの映像資料の最も素晴らしい点であり、新しい学習効果が期待できます。動画で最初に Bad Dialogue、次に Good Dialogue を見て比較してください。内容把握、映像、言語などの視点から場面全体を理解し、総合的にとらえ、下の設問に答えてみてください。Play Both を繰り返し見れば、次第に細部にも注意がいきとどき、楽しみながら自然に英語のリスニング力もつくでしょう。

また、この映像学習はまた日本の看護の場面との差異に興味を持って見ていけば、立派な異文化理解にもつながることでしょう。

III Comprehension Check

Good Dialogue の内容理解を確認するための音声のみの設問と、選択肢から選ぶ解答から成っています。英語の質問を理解できるかどうかが鍵となりますから、質問文を正確に聞き取れたかどうかを確認するために、この部分の書き取りをお勧めします。次第に聞き取りが上達することが感じられて励みになることでしょう。

IV Complete the Dialogue

今度は Good Dialogue を聞きながらスクリプトの一部の空欄を埋めていく活動です。最初は英語のスピードに慣れるまで苦労する人もいるでしょうが、自分が苦手とする部分が明らかになり、画面の状況や動作と合わせて会話を理解できるようになり、生きた会話を経験できるでしょう。ユニットが進むにつれ英語のリズムにも慣れ、速く話される個所も聞き取りましょう。

ここまでは、かなりの程度を自宅学習とし、クラスで答えを確認する授業方法も考えられます。少しゆっくりとしたスピードで吹き替え収録をした教室用音声 CD もご利用ください。

V Substitution Practice

使用頻度の高い構文の一部を置き換える練習です。自然に英語が話せるまでリラックスして練習しましょう。

Ⅵ Expand Your Vocabulary

語彙を豊富にする練習問題ですが、スペリングも重要です。宿題とするのもよいでしょう。

Ⅶ Speaking Practice

クラスでの言語活動の中心となる会話練習です。指示に従って役割を交代したり、場面を変えたりして、コミュニケーションを楽しみましょう。決して、ただ暗記してそれを話すのではなく、相手の反応を見ながら自分の感情や思いをコミュニケーションにこめて話してみましょう。

いろいろな表現を覚えましょう

ユニットの内容に関連する重要な表現を集めてみました。臨床の場面ですぐ使用可能なものですので、レベルに応じて様々に使用してください。また、卒業後、看護の現場で必要なときに参考にしてください。

資料・コラム

会話教材ではカバーしにくい医療系教育の基礎となる体の部位、コミュニケーション・スキル、医療系の用語などを集めたものです。会話と同様に重要な部分なので、レベルに合わせて活用して欲しいと願っております。

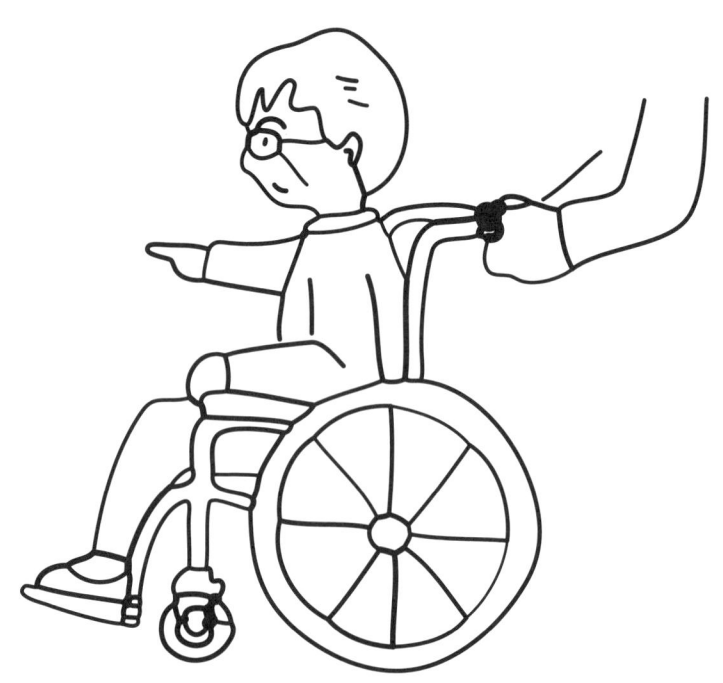

Contents

Unit 1 Greetings 1
  [語彙：医療従事者]

Unit 2 Giving Explanations 7
  [体の外部図・名称]

Unit 3 Tests (X-ray) 13
  [体の頭部・名称]

Unit 4 Inviting the Patient to Talk, and Listening 19
  [体の内部図・名称]

Unit 5 Nursing Care and Asking Permission 25
  [語彙：看護処置用品]

Unit 6 Injection 31
  [語彙・表現：感染症と予防接種]

Unit 7 Vital Signs 37
  [体温・体重・身長の換算]

Unit 8 Rehabilitation and Asking Questions 43
  [Important Communication Skills in Nursing]

Unit 9 Operation 49
  [健康に関することわざ]

Unit 10 Positioning the Patient and Giving Instructions 55
  [Pain Scale]

Unit 11 Medication 61
  [語彙：疾病と創傷（1）]

Unit 12 Discharge and Goodbye 67
  [語彙：疾病と創傷（2）]

Unit 13 Negotiation Management 73
  [Tips for Nursing Communication]

Unit 14 Consultation (Pregnancy) 79
  [語彙：看護・医療用品]

Unit 15 Consultation (Cancer) 85
  [Common Abbreviations]

Student ID No. _____ Name _____

Unit 1
Greetings

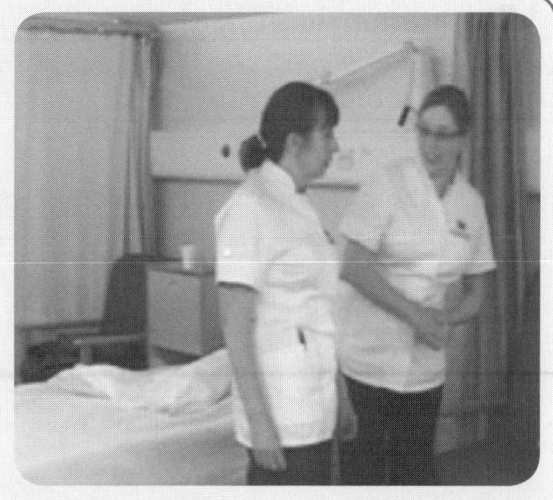

自然でさわやかな挨拶は友好的なコミュニケーションのスタートとなります。時、場所、場合を考えて挨拶を交わしてみましょう。

I Key Sentences

Check the sentences below, and read them aloud to memorize them.

1. I'd like to introduce you to your doctor.
2. This is Jean Brown.
3. It's nice to meet you.
4. I'll look after you during your time in the hospital.
5. We'll see you later. Bye-bye.

II Improve Your Communication Skills Play Both

Watch the bad and good dialogues, and answer the following questions.

1. the good dialogue ではどのように改善されたでしょうか。
2. 両方のクリップを見て、挨拶の役割は何か、また相手によって変わるかどうかを話し合ってみましょう。
3. 看護の場でのコミュニケーションではどのようなことが大切かを、具体的に各自書き出してみましょう。

III Comprehension Check

Watch the good dialogue and choose the most appropriate answer to each question on the DVD.

1. **Q:** [   ]
   a. In the evening   **b.** In the morning   **c.** Yesterday morning

2. **Q:** [   ]
   a. Jean Smith   **b.** Mr. Smith   **c.** Jean Brown

3. **Q:** [   ]
   a. He is sitting on the chair near the bed.
   b. He is reading a book in bed.
   c. He is in bed waiting for the nurses to come.

4. **Q:** [   ]
   a. The head nurse
   b. A male nurse who was not in the room
   c. The nurse who introduced the head nurse to the patient

IV Complete the Dialogue

Watch the good dialogue again and fill in the blanks.

(N1: Nurse N2: Nurse P: Patient)

N1:   Hello, Jean. I'd like (1)_____ _____ you to Mr. Smith.

N2:   OK.

N1:   (2)_____ _____ _____ _____.

N2:   Fine.

N1:   (3)_____ _____ _____. Hello, Mr. Smith.

P: Morning, morning.

N1:   Good morning. I would like to introduce you to our head nurse. This is Jean Brown.

N2: Hello, Mr. Smith. (4)___ ___ ___?

P: Hello, I'm very well, thank you.

N2: (5)___.

P: Nice to meet you.

N1: She's going to be looking after you during your time in hospital.

P: Good.

N2: So if there's anything that (6)___ ___, don't hesitate to call me.

P: No, thank.... I, (7)___ ___. Thank you. Thank you very much.

N1: OK.

P: Thank you.

N1: We'll (8)___ ___ ___.

N2: Bye-bye.

V Substitution Practice

Replace the shaded expressions with those below and read them aloud.

1. I'm Yoko Sato, **your primary nurse**.
   - a student nurse
   - a surgeon
   - a pharmacist
   - a sophomore at _____ College/University

2. A: **This is** your doctor, Mr. Kato.
   - Let me introduce
   - I'd like to introduce

   Kato: How do you do?

   C: How do you do? **It's nice** to meet you.
   - I'm glad
   - I'm pleased

3. A: How do you feel?
   B: Not so well, I'm afraid.
      I feel uneasy about my condition
      I feel comfortable

4. Don't hesitate to ask me any questions.
                to call the nurse
                to come to the nurse station

VI Expand Your Vocabulary

From the box below, choose and write down the English words with the same meaning as the following Japanese words.

看護師 _____   准看護師 _____

看護助手 _____   看護部長 _____

訪問看護師 _____   専門看護師 _____

保健師 _____   看護実習生 _____

院長 _____   事務長 _____

> clinical nurse specialist (CNS)   chief administrator
> hospital director   director of the nursing department
> visiting nurse   registered nurse (RN)
> nurse's aide   licensed practical nurse (LPN)
> student nurse   public health nurse

VII Speaking Practice

1. the good dialogueを見て自分で練習して覚えましょう。
2. 次に3人で教科書を見ないで会話してみましょう。
3. お互いに自己紹介をし、自分のことについて自由に会話をしてみましょう。

Unit 1　Greetings

いろいろな表現を覚えましょう

☞ **1.　出会いの挨拶**

A: Hello/ Hi/ Good morning/ Good afternoon/ Good evening, Mr. White.
　　How are you? (How are things?/ How's it going?)
B: Quite well, thank you, and you?

注：出来るなら、最初はMr.(Mrs., Miss, Ms.) Smith のように姓を呼び、相手からPlease call me John. などと言われてから名を呼ぶのがよいでしょう。

☞ **2.　再会の挨拶**

I haven't seen you for a long time.
You are quite a stranger.
Long time no see.

☞ **3.　別れの挨拶**

See you later/ again/ tomorrow/ next month.
Goodbye. Bye.
Have a nice day.
Good day. Good night.
I'll come back soon.
I'll come to see you again this afternoon.

☞ **4.　患者さんを安心させる表現**

Don't worry.
There's no need to worry.
I quite understand you are a bit uneasy now.
I'll do my best to take good care of you.
I'll try to make your stay as comfortable as possible.

語彙: Hospital Personnel 医療従事者

1. Administrators 管理職
   - hospital director 院長
   - director of the nursing department 看護部長
   - chief administrator 事務長

2. Nursing Department 看護部
   - supervisor 管理師長
   - clinical nurse specialist (CNS) 専門看護師
   - registered nurse (RN) 看護師
   - licensed practical nurse (LPN) 准看護師
   - nurse's aide; nursing assistant 看護助手
   - student nurse 看護実習生
   - visiting nurse 訪問看護師
   - public health nurse 保健師
   - head nurse (nurse in charge) 主任看護師
   - primary nurse プライマリーナース

3. Staff スタッフ
   - pharmacist 薬剤師
   - medical social worker ソーシャルワーカー
   - lab technician 臨床検査技師
   - X-ray technician X線技師
   - dietitian, nutritionist 栄養士
   - physical therapist (PT) 理学療法士
   - occupational therapist (OT) 作業療法士
   - speech therapist 言語療法士
   - orthoptist 視能訓練士
   - clinical psychologist 臨床心理士
   - clerk (secretary) 事務職員
   - cashier 会計係
   - receptionist 受付係
   - emergency medical technician (EMT) 救急医療隊員

4. Physicians 医師
   - resident 研修医
   - internist 内科医
   - cardiologist 循環器専門医
   - gastroenterologist 消化器専門医
   - pulmonologist 呼吸器専門医
   - surgeon 外科医
   - orthopedist 整形外科医
   - gynecologist 婦人科医
   - obstetrician 産科医
   - pediatrician 小児科医
   - psychiatrist 精神科医
   - neurologist 神経科医
   - urologist 泌尿器科医
   - dentist 歯科医
   - dermatologist 皮膚科医
   - anesthesiologist 麻酔医
   - radiologist 放射線医
   - ophthalmologist, eye doctor 眼科医
   - otorhinolaryngologist
     = ENT (ear, nose, throat doctor) 耳鼻咽喉科医

Unit 2
Giving Explanations

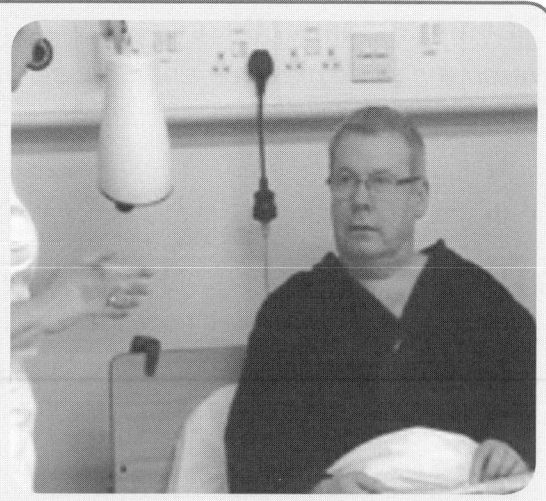

どのような点に配慮したら、相手が説明を理解しそれに従って行動できるか、映像をよく観察して考えてみましょう。

Ⅰ Key Sentences

Check the sentences below, and read them aloud to memorize them.

1. I'm going to explain the schedule for tomorrow.
2. The doctor will be round to see you at eleven.
3. Lunchtime will be at twelve.
4. We'll come and give you a bed-bath.
5. OK. That's good.

Ⅱ Improve Your Communication Skills　　WEB動画　DVD　Play Both

Watch the bad and good dialogues, and answer the following questions.

1. the good dialogue ではどんな点が改善されたでしょうか。
2. 説明はどのように始めて、どのような説明の仕方が良いと思いましたか。

III Comprehension Check

Watch the good dialogue and choose the most appropriate answer to each question on the DVD.

1. **Q:** [   ]
    a. At 8 o'clock   b. At 7 o'clock   c. At 6 o'clock

2. **Q:** [   ]
    a. He feels it's necessary.   b. He feels it's quite good to know about it.
    c. He's not interested in the hospital schedule at all.

3. **Q:** [   ]
    a. In bed in his room   b. In the treatment room
    c. In the bathroom

4. **Q:** [   ]
    a. Before lunch   b. In the evening   c. After lunch

IV Complete the Dialogue

Watch the good dialogue again and fill in the blanks.

(N: Nurse P: Patient)

N: Good morning, Mr. Smith, how are you?

P: Morning. Oh, I'm OK, thank you.

N: That's good. I just wanted to explain (1)_____ _____ _____ _____ for today.

P: All right, yes.

N: OK. Ah, 7 o'clock, it will be (2)_____ _____.

P: OK.

N: And (3)_____ _____, the doctors will be round to see you.

P: OK, that's good, good, good.

N: And then lunchtime at 12.

P: Right.

Unit 2 Giving Explanations

N: OK, it's good to know (4)_____ _____ _____ _____, I think.

P: (5)_____.

N: Ah, about 11, if you (6)_____ _____ _____ _____, we'll come and (7)_____ _____ _____ _____. Is that OK?

P: Oh, um…yes, yes, yes, that's fine, thank you.

N: It will make you feel (8)_____ _____ before your lunch.

P: Yes. I imagine, yeah.

N: (9)_____ _____ _____ _____.

P: No, no, that's fine. Thank you, thank you very much.

N: OK. I'll see you later.

P: OK.

V Substitution Practice

Replace the shaded expressions with those below and read them aloud.

1. I'd like to explain about the hospital schedule .
   - the registration
   - the consent form
   - the coming operation

2. The visiting hours in this hospital are from 5:00 p.m. to 8:00 p.m. on weekdays .
   - from 1:00 p.m. to 8:00 p.m. on weekends
   - from 10:00 a.m. to 12:00 noon on the day of operation

3. I'll come and give you a bed-bath .
   - a foot-bath
   - a massage
   - medicine
   - a brochure

4. If you feel up to [it / a foot-bath / taking a walk / a shampoo / sitting up], please call me again.

5. OK, that's [fine / right / good / wonderful / quite nice / not so bad].

VI Expand Your Vocabulary

From the box below, choose and write down the English words with the same meaning as the following Japanese words.

入院受付 _____   面会時間 _____

消灯 _____   個室 _____

ナースステーション _____   起床時間 _____

洗面台 _____   ロッカー _____

談話室 _____   診察室 _____

```
lights-out          patients' lounge      wake-up time
private room        sink                  nurses' station
consultation room   locker                visiting hours
admission office
```

VII Speaking Practice

1. the good dialogueを見て自分で練習してよく覚えましょう。
2. ペアになり役割を交代して練習しましょう。
3. The daily schedule あるいは Visiting rules について説明してみましょう。

Unit 2　Giving Explanations

いろいろな表現を覚えましょう

☞　**1．病室での説明**

Please read this guide/pamphlet/leaflet.
Please change into this hospital gown.
The nurse call bell is here by the pillow.
You can keep your things in the closet.
Here's a towel for you.
Dinner is served at six in the big dining room.
This sign shows the emergency escape route.

☞　**2．説明の確認を得る表現**

Let me talk to you about our care plan for you.
The doctor is going to explain about the surgery.
Has the doctor told you about your operation?
Were you satisfied with the explanation?
Could you understand the explanation about your illness?

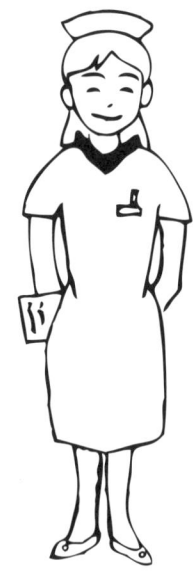

体の外部図・名称

体の部位を表す英語を、下の英語群から選んで（　　）内に書き入れましょう。

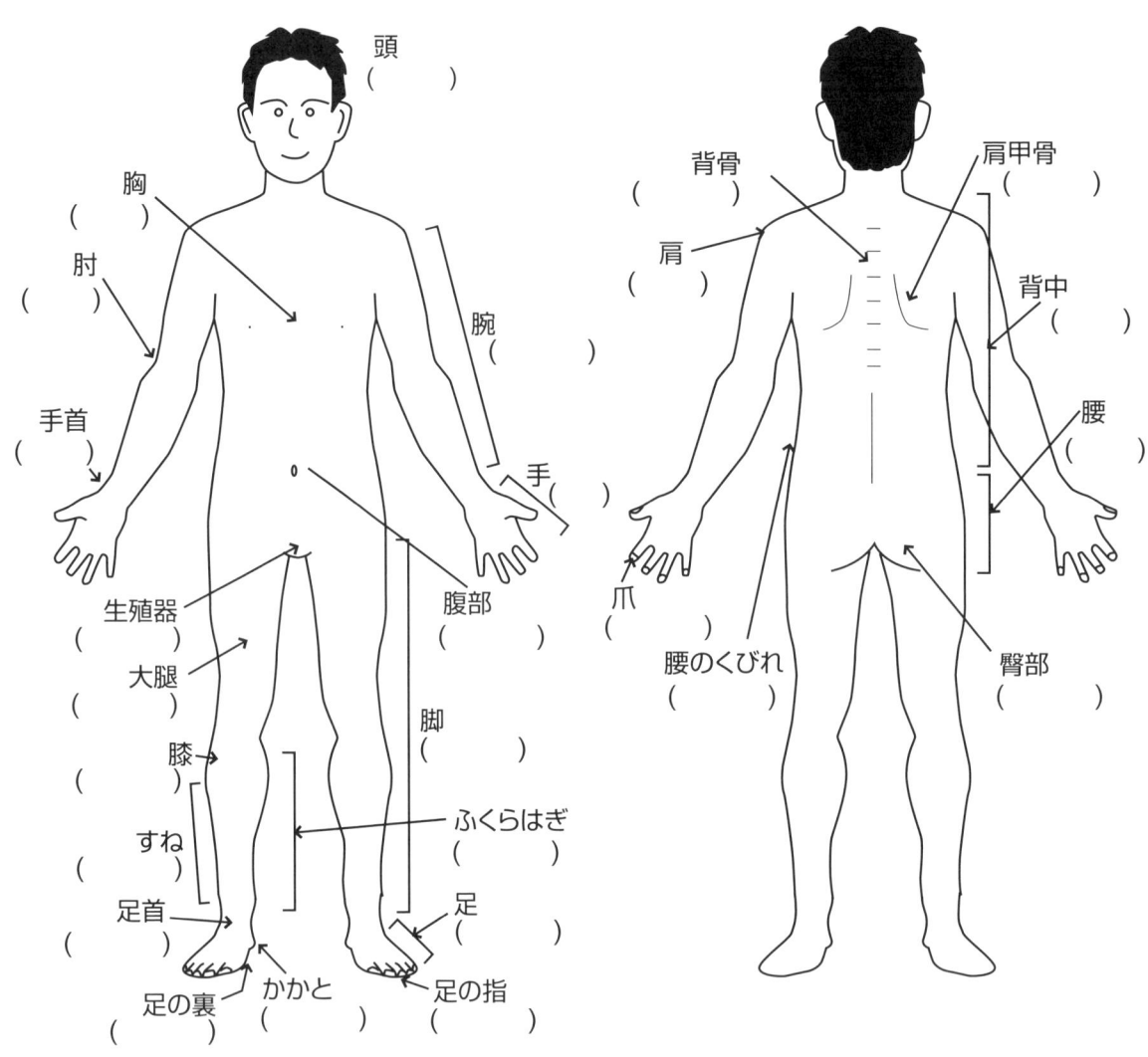

a) abdomen　　b) ankle　　c) arm　　d) buttocks
e) lower back　f) (upper) back　g) calf　h) chest
i) elbow　　　j) shoulder　　k) genitals　l) hand
m) head　　　n) heel　　　　o) knee　　　p) leg
q) nail　　　　r) shin　　　　s) shoulder blade　t) sole
u) spine　　　v) thigh　　　w) foot　　　x) toe(s)
y) waist　　　z) wrist

Unit 3
Tests (X-ray)

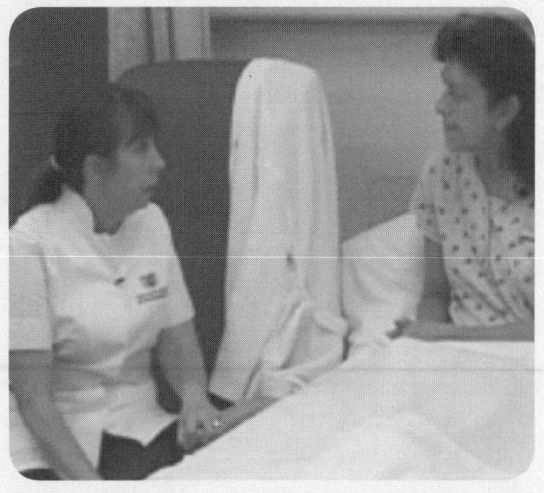

検査は病気とその症状に合わせて種類も多いので、患者さんに的確に伝えることが重要です。患者さんになったつもりで質問してみましょう。

I Key Sentences

Check the sentences below, and read them aloud to memorize them.

1. Have you ever had a chest X-ray?
2. I had a chest X-ray five years ago.
3. We need to do another one tomorrow.
4. Somebody will be coming to take you.
5. I'll take you down to the X-ray department.

II Improve Your Communication Skills　　Play Both

Watch the bad and good dialogues, and answer the following questions.

1. the good dialogue ではどのように改善されたでしょうか。
2. the good dialogueで 'somebody' が使用されていますが、患者さんはどのように感じると思いますか。また、他にどのような表現が考えられますか。

III Comprehension Check

Watch the good dialogue and choose the most appropriate answer to each question on the DVD.

1. **Q:** [   ]
   - **a.** Very serious
   - **b.** Excellent
   - **c.** Not so bad

2. **Q:** [   ]
   - **a.** Tomorrow morning
   - **b.** The next day
   - **c.** This morning

3. **Q:** [   ]
   - **a.** Another nurse
   - **b.** Somebody the nurse asked
   - **c.** The nurse herself

4. **Q:** [   ]
   - **a.** Less than one hour
   - **b.** About one hour
   - **c.** A few hours

IV Complete the Dialogue

Watch the good dialogue again and fill in the blanks.

(N: Nurse P: Patient)

N: Hello, Mary.

P: Hello.

N: (1)_____ _____ _____?

P: I'm (2)_____ _____ _____.

N: Good. (3)_____ _____ _____ _____ a chest X-ray?

P: Um, yes, I have. Um, about (4)_____ _____ _____.

N: Ten years ago. (5)_____ _____ to do another one this morning. So somebody will be (6)_____ _____ about (7)_____ _____ _____ _____ to take you down to (8)_____ _____ _____. Is that OK?

P: Yes, thank you.

N: OK.

14

Unit 3 Tests (X-ray)

V Substitution Practice

Replace the shaded expressions with those below and read them aloud.

1. Have you ever had [an ECG (electrocardiogram)] ?
   - a cardiac catheterization
   - an endoscopy examination
   - a hearing test

2. When did you have [an X-ray] ?
   - a CT (computerized tomography) scan
   - a health check
   - a mammography

3. The results should be ready by [next Monday].
   - noon
   - next Friday
   - April 12
   - the 23rd of September

4. You need to provide [a urine sample] for testing.
   - a stool sample
   - a sputum sample
   - a blood sample

VI Expand Your Vocabulary

From the box below, choose and write down the English words with the same meaning as the following Japanese words.

検尿 _____   検便 _____

脳波 _____   喀痰標本 _____

生検 _____   蛋白質 _____

追跡検査 _____   検査室 _____

血糖 _____   （血液、尿などを）採集する _____

blood sugar	urine test	brain wave
protein	follow-up examination	collect
stool test	sputum sample	biopsy
laboratory		

15

VII Speaking Practice

1. the good dialogueを見て自分で練習してよく覚えましょう。
2. ペアになって役割を交代して練習しましょう。
3. 患者さんと看護師になって、次のような質問に対して答える会話を行ってみましょう。

    Why do I need an X-ray?   What will it show?
    How long will it take?   Will it hurt?
    Will I be undressed?

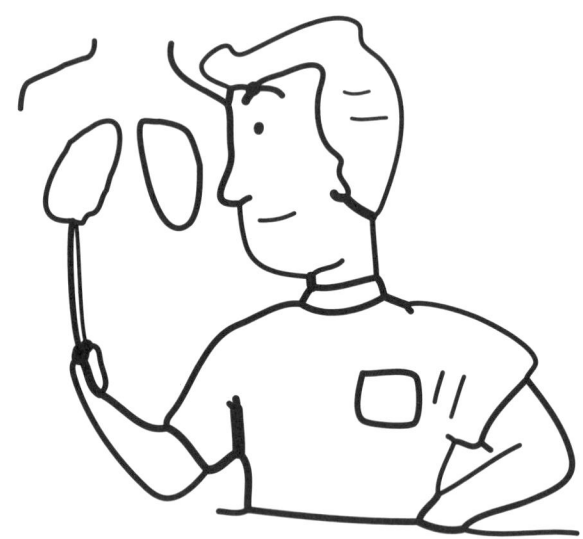

Unit 3　Tests (X-ray)

いろいろな表現を覚えましょう

☞ **1．検査標本の採り方に関する表現**

採血
Please hold out your left arm and make a fist.
I am going to collect some of your blood, 8cc (cubic centimeters).

尿検査
Please fill about one-third of this cup with urine.
Please first urinate a small amount into the toilet, and then fill the cup.
Please leave the cup on the shelf in the toilet.
It will be tested for sugar, protein and other substances.

検便
Please bring a stool specimen in this container.
Insert this glass stick into your rectum, and then take it out.

胃の検査
Try not to belch, please.
Drink a mouthful of barium, please.
Please drink the laxative to expel the barium.

☞ **2．その他の表現**

The doctor has ordered an ultrasonography.

Let's get ready to go for your PET (positron-emission tomography) scan.

Please remove any accessories/ metallic objects.

You can keep your underwear on.

The test will take about 40 minutes.

Please close your eyes lightly during the exam.

体の頭部・名称

頭部の部位を表す英語を、下の英語群から選んで(　　)内に書き入れましょう。

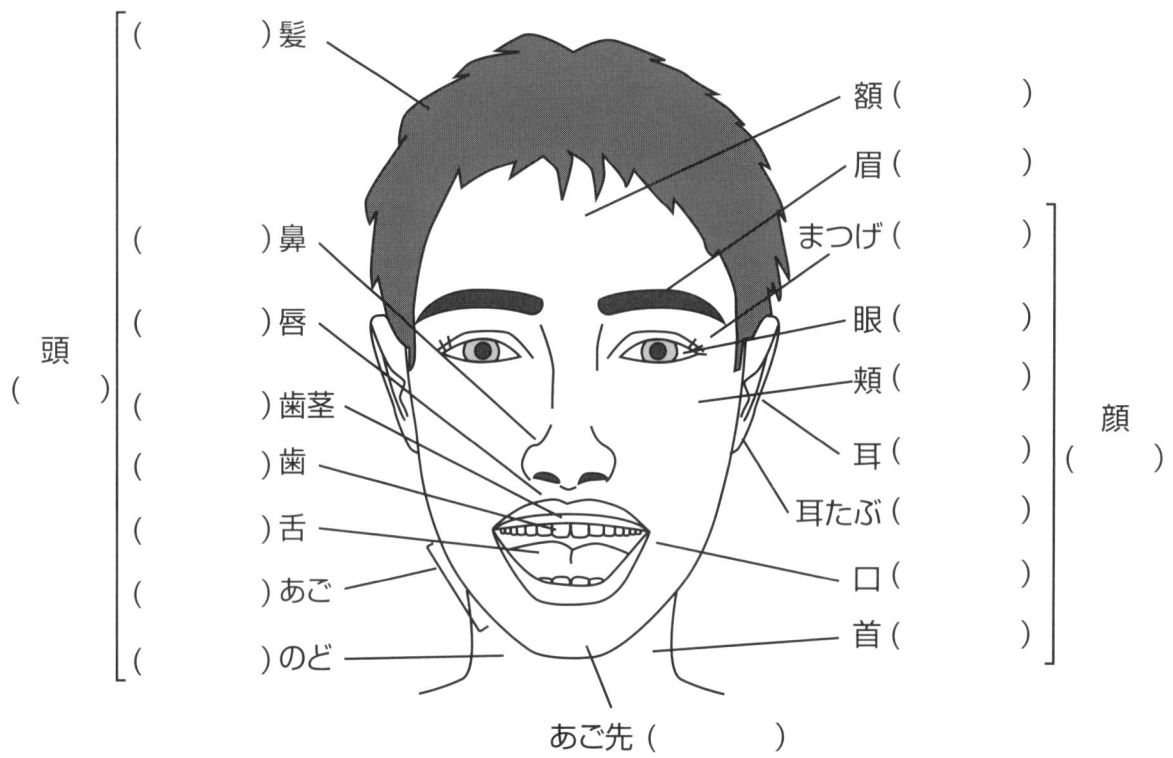

- a) cheek
- b) chin
- c) ear
- d) earlobe
- e) eye
- f) eyebrow
- g) eyelashes
- h) forehead
- i) gums
- j) hair
- k) head
- l) jaw
- m) lips
- n) mouth
- o) neck
- p) nose
- q) teeth
- r) throat
- s) tongue
- t) face

手指の名称

英語で親指はthumbと呼ばれ、fingersの中には入りません。人差し指はforefinger, index finger, first fingerと呼ばれ、中指はmiddle finger, second finger、薬指はring finger, third finger、小指はlittle finger, pinkie（米口語）となります。

Unit 4
Inviting the Patient to Talk, and Listening

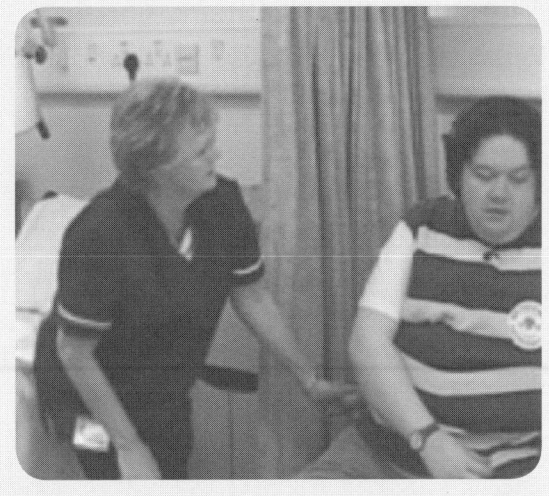

関心や共感を示しながら、患者さんに発言を促し傾聴しましょう。時には恐れや不安、怒りなど個人的な状況や感情も酌みとってあげましょう。

I Key Sentences

Check the sentences below, and read them aloud to memorize them.

1. You look a bit worried.
2. I can't get to my cup.
3. Here we are. This is your good hand, isn't it?
4. Is there something else bothering you?
5. We'll listen and we'll come when you press the bell.

II Improve Your Communication Skills Play Both

Watch the bad and good dialogues, and answer the following questions.

1. the good dialogue ではどのように改善されたでしょうか
2. 看護では傾聴は重要なことですが、傾聴していることを患者さんに伝えるにはどのようにしたらいいと思いますか。
3. 看護の現場での傾聴が困難な場合の原因を探ってみましょう。

III Comprehension Check

Watch the good dialogue and choose the most appropriate answer to each question on the DVD.

1. **Q:** [   ]
   a. Because he asks her to come.   b. Because he looks worried.
   c. Because he looks angry.

2. **Q:** [   ]
   a. He can't reach the nurse call button.
   b. He can't press the buzzer.
   c. The nurse didn't come quickly.

3. **Q:** [   ]
   a. His right hand   b. His left hand

4. **Q:** [   ]
   a. It is not appropriate to this situation.   b. It is not polite enough.
   c. It is polite and quick.

IV Complete the Dialogue

Watch the good dialogue again and fill in the blanks.

(N: Nurse P: Patient)

N: Hello, Charles. You're looking....

P: Hello, Lynne.

N: Hello. You look really (1)_____. Are you all right?

P: I...I can't get to my buzzer.

N: Oh, (2)_____ _____ put on the wrong side, hasn't it? Here we are. Look, this is your good hand, isn't it?

P: Yeah.

N: Do you want to (3)_____ it there?

P: Yeah.

N: And then if you need us, you can press the bell. Was there something else (4)_____ _____?

P: When I want to (5)_____ _____ _____ _____, and I press the bell, will someone come quickly?

N: Yes, they will, yes, they will. I'll make sure that somebody comes as soon as (6)_____ _____ _____ _____. All right?

P: I don't…I don't want to (7)_____ _____ _____.

N: No, (8)_____ _____ _____ _____. We'll…we'll listen and we'll come when you ring.

P: OK.

N: All right. OK.

V Substitution Practice

Replace the shaded expressions with those below and read them aloud.

1. You look really tired .
   - well
   - nice
   - normal
   - pale
   - anxious

2. Do you want to rest the bell on the bed ?
   - put it on the desk
   - keep it in the bedside table
   - hang it in the closet

3. Somebody will come as soon as you press the bell.
   - The head nurse
   - The doctor on duty
   - The staff

4. We'll listen and come when you ring .
   - when you press the buzzer
   - when you call us
   - when you need us

VI Expand Your Vocabulary

From the box below, choose and write down the English words with the same meaning as the following Japanese words.

悩ます _____   押す _____

（ベルを）鳴らす _____   傾聴する _____

置く _____   トイレ _____

事故（おもらし）_____   緊急事態 _____

率直に _____   遠慮なく話す _____

```
    accident              listen to              press
    emergency             speak out              toilet
    put                   worry                  ring
    frankly
```

VII Speaking Practice

1. the good dialogueを見て自分で練習してよく覚えましょう。
2. ペアになり役割を交代して練習しましょう。
3. 傾聴がうまくいかなかった場合、患者さんとの間でどのようなことが起こる可能性があるか話し合ってみましょう。

いろいろな表現を覚えましょう

☞ **1. 患者さんに話しかける表現**

Is something the matter? Is anything wrong?

Is there anything worrying/ bothering you?

☞ **2. 患者さんが訴える表現**

I was very worried about my headache.

It upset me when the doctor told me about the operation.

It made me cry when I had that sharp pain.

Nobody knew what was wrong with my eye.

☞ **3. 患者さんを元気づける表現**

You look great!   You can make it.   Don't worry.

You did very well.   You did a good job.   Stop complaining.

☞ **4. 状況の変化を知らせる表現**

Please let us know if you begin to feel sick.

Please go to the restroom beforehand.

It will be over soon/ in a few hours.

I'm finished now.

You can start taking baths from today.

You can eat a regular diet after that.

Please come to the treatment room at once.

Please calm down and wait for the doctor.

体の内部図・名称

体の内部の臓器を表す英語に相当する日本語を、下の日本語群から選んで（　　）内に記入しましょう。

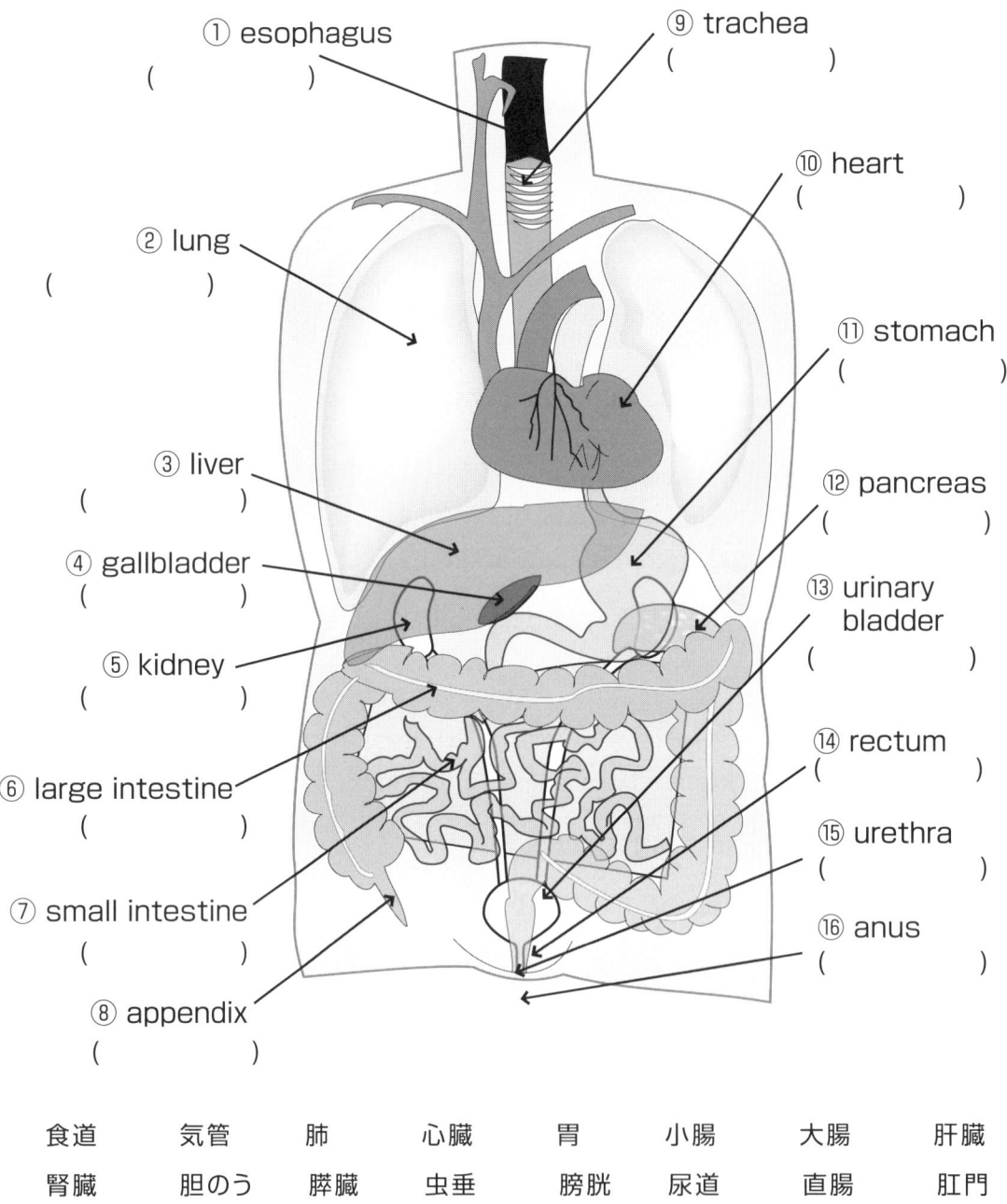

① esophagus （　　　　）
② lung （　　　　）
③ liver （　　　　）
④ gallbladder （　　　　）
⑤ kidney （　　　　）
⑥ large intestine （　　　　）
⑦ small intestine （　　　　）
⑧ appendix （　　　　）
⑨ trachea （　　　　）
⑩ heart （　　　　）
⑪ stomach （　　　　）
⑫ pancreas （　　　　）
⑬ urinary bladder （　　　　）
⑭ rectum （　　　　）
⑮ urethra （　　　　）
⑯ anus （　　　　）

食道　　気管　　肺　　心臓　　胃　　小腸　　大腸　　肝臓
腎臓　　胆のう　　膵臓　　虫垂　　膀胱　　尿道　　直腸　　肛門

Unit 5
Nursing Care and Asking Permission

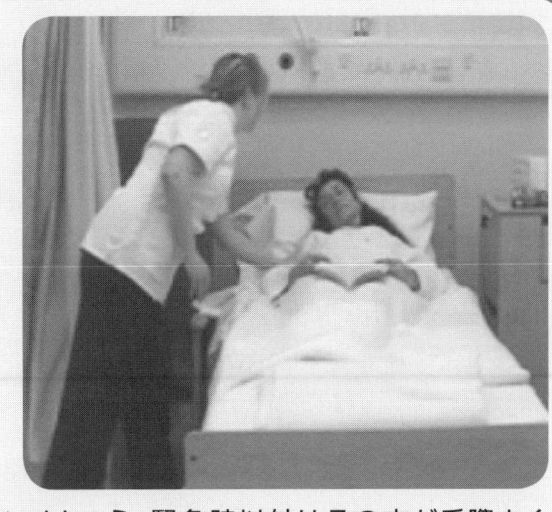

患者さんの許可を得てから看護行為を行いましょう。緊急時以外はその方が手際よく処置でき、患者さんも協力してくれるでしょう。

I Key Sentences

Check the sentences below, and read them aloud to memorize them.

1. I hear things went well.
2. I'm sorry to wake you up.
3. I hope to have a look at your wound.
4. Let's just close the curtain so you have more privacy.
5. Shall I put your towel back here?

II Improve Your Communication Skills   Play Both

Watch the bad and good dialogues, and answer the following questions.

1. the good dialogueではどのような点が改善されたでしょうか。
2. 特に、the good dialogueでの看護師の態度に関して感じたことがあれば、その理由を述べなさい。

III Comprehension Check

Watch the good dialogue and choose the most appropriate answer to each question on the DVD.

1. **Q:** [   ]
   a. Reading a magazine   b. Listening to music   c. Sleeping

2. **Q:** [   ]
   a. To see her face   b. To change the dressing
   c. To tell her about the operation

3. **Q:** [   ]
   a. Because the nurse wakes her up.
   b. Because the doctor hasn't come to the room with her.
   c. Because the nurse disturbs her while she is reading a book.

4. **Q:** [   ]
   a. She rolls up her sleeves.   b. She helps the patient stand up.
   c. She closes the curtain.

IV Complete the Dialogue

Watch the good dialogue again and fill in the blanks.

(N: Nurse P: Patient)

N: Mary?

P: Hmm?

N: Hello, Mary. Hello.

　　 I hear (1)_____ _____ _____ _____.

P: Mm-hmm.

N: Are you (2)_____?

P: Mm.

N: (3)_____ _____ _____ to wake you. I was hoping to have a

　　 look at (4)_____ _____. Is that OK?

P: Mm.

N: OK, and would it be all right if I (5)_____ _____ _____?

P: OK, yes.

N: So can I just do that now?

P: Yes.

N: (6)_____ _____ _____ your book? OK. Let's just (7)_____ _____ so you have (8)_____ _____ _____ _____.

OK, let me just help you sit up. (9)_____. Can I just…OK?

V Substitution Practice

Replace the shaded expressions with those below and read them aloud.

1. | I hear | things went very well.
   | I know |
   | We hear |
   | I noticed |
   | They knew |

2. I'm very sorry | to wake you |.
   | to make you feel uncomfortable |
   | to make you sad |
   | to have kept you waiting |

3. Would it be all right if I looked at | your wound |?
   | your bedsore |
   | this intravenous drip |
   | the ice pillow |
   | the inhaler |

4. Shall I | take your book |?
   | turn off the TV |
   | turn on the radio |
   | fill in the form for you |

VI Expand Your Vocabulary

From the box below, choose and write down the English words with the same meaning as the following Japanese words.

プライバシー _____   倫理 _____

点滴痕 _____   絆創膏 _____

患者の権利 _____   保護する _____

切開（手術）_____   湿布 _____

消毒する _____   止血する _____

> compress   adhesive tape   protect
> incision   stop the bleeding   ethics
> privacy   patients' rights   disinfect
> IV site

VII Speaking Practice

1. the good dialogueを見て自分で練習してよく覚えましょう。
2. ペアになり役割を交代して練習しましょう。
3. 看護師と患者になり、pulse, blood pressure, temperatureを測る前に、患者さんの許可を得る会話をしてみましょう。

Unit 5 Nursing Care and Asking Permission

いろいろな表現を覚えましょう

☞ 1. 患者さんに提案をする表現

Why don't you go for a walk outside?
How about asking the doctor when he comes round?
How about a cup of coffee now?
You could switch on the TV.

☞ 2. 処置に関する表現

I am going to put on the ointment.
I'll give you a suppository. Please insert it into the anus.
I am going to give you an enema.
I'll press out the pus.
Please apply this lotion to the area.
Please put in eye drops.

☞ 3. 看護計画などに関する用語

nursing interview [NI]
nursing diagnosis [ND]
nursing process
    1. assessment
    2. planning
    3. implementation
    4. evaluation
SOAP charting
    1. subjective data [S]
    2. objective data [O]
    3. assessment [A]
    4. plan [P]
nursing-care plan [NP]   therapeutic plan [TP]
educational plan [EP]   progress note [PN]
quality control [QC]   patient-nurse interaction [Pt-N-I]

語彙：看護処置用品

absorbent cotton; cotton balls	脱脂綿	latex gloves	ラテックス手袋
adhesive bandage; adhesive tape	絆創膏	lukewarm water	ぬるま湯
antiseptic solution	消毒薬	needle	注射針
condom; rubber	コンドーム	oiled paper	油紙
cotton swab; Q-tip, applicator	綿棒	paper diaper	紙おむつ
disinfectant	殺菌(消毒)剤	sling	吊り包帯, 三角巾
endoscope	内視鏡	surgical gown/cap/mask	手術用着衣・帽子・マスク
gauze	ガーゼ		
hearing aid	補聴器	test tube	試験管
ice bag/pillow	氷嚢, 氷枕	tweezers; small forceps	ピンセット

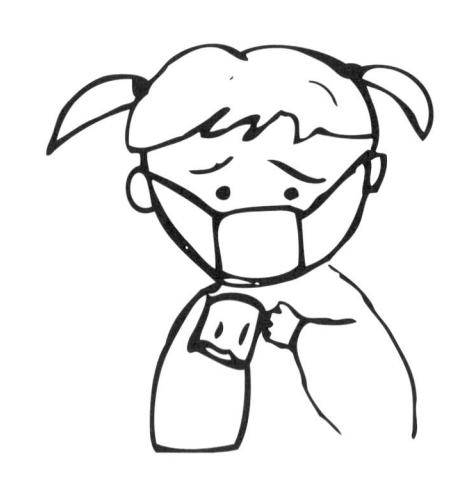

Unit 6
Injection

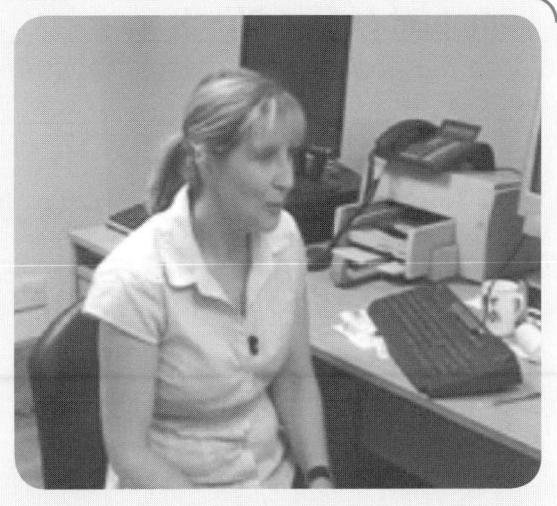

日本でも看護師が注射をする機会が多くなってきています。その前後の指示表現をよく覚え、スムーズに進行させましょう。

I Key Sentences

Check the sentences below, and read them aloud to memorize them.

1. I'm off on holiday (vacation).
2. You're going to have a tetanus injection.
3. I'm going to swab the wound.
4. Are you agreeable to have it?
5. Can you roll up your sleeve on your left arm?

II Improve Your Communication Skills — Play Both

Watch the bad and good dialogues, and answer the following questions.

1. the good dialogueではどのような点が改善されていましたか。
2. 注射をするときの会話は簡潔な方がいいか、それとも十分な会話が必要でしょうか。

III Comprehension Check

Watch the good dialogue and choose the most appropriate answer to each question on the DVD.

1. **Q:** [   ]
   a. To the hospital   **b.** To Spain   **c.** To Italy

2. **Q:** [   ]
   a. To consult about his long trip   **b.** To have a tetanus injection
   c. To have a health checkup

3. **Q:** [   ]
   a. It's on the shelf.   **b.** It's on her desk.   **c.** It's in the box.

4. **Q:** [   ]
   a. She does nothing.   **b.** She swabs his arm.
   c. She pats him on the right arm.

IV Complete the Dialogue

Watch the good dialogue again and fill in the blanks.

(N: Nurse P: Patient)

N:　　So you're (1)_____ _____ _____.

P:　　Yeah, Spain.

N:　　(2)_____ _____ you haven't had a tetanus (3)_____ for a while.

P:　　Mm-hmm.

N:　　Well, (4)_____ _____ one ready for you here. Are you agreeable (5)_____ _____ it? Today?

P:　　Yes, yes.

N:　　Lovely, OK. Can you (6)_____ _____ your sleeve a little bit on this arm?

P:　　Yeah, sure.

N: OK, I'm just going to (7)_____.

P: OK.

N: I've got it (8)_____. OK? Sharp prick coming.

P: OK.

V Substitution Practice

Replace the shaded expressions with those below and read them aloud.

1. Have you had a vaccination for diphtheria ?
   - polio
   - influenza
   - cholera
   - chickenpox

2. Do you agree to have a shot ?
   - open the curtain
   - have surgery
   - change your dressing

3. Can you roll up your sleeve ?
   - touch your knees
   - turn around
   - raise your shirt

4. I'm giving the injection in your thigh .
   - abdomen
   - shoulder
   - hip

VI Expand Your Vocabulary

From the box below, choose and write down the English words with the same meaning as the following Japanese words.

注射針 _____   点滴 _____

皮下注射 _____   静脈注射 _____

筋肉注射 _____   予防接種 _____

(チクリと)刺す _____ (綿棒で)ふく _____

痛む _____   我慢する _____

```
  swab            vein injection        intravenous drip
  prick           needle                muscular injection
  stand           vaccination           hypodermic injection
  hurt
```

VII Speaking Practice

1. the good dialogueを見て自分で練習してよく覚えましょう。
2. ペアになり役割を交代して練習しましょう。
3. 注射や包帯をするときに、どの程度患者さんに話すか実際にやってみましょう。

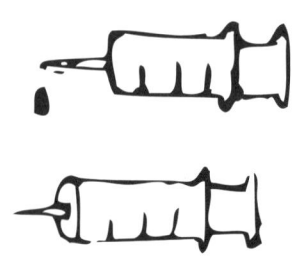

Unit 6　Injection

いろいろな表現を覚えましょう

☞　**1.　注射の前後の注意に関する表現**

Please relax.　　　　　Relax your muscle.
Don't be afraid.
This won't hurt.　　　This may hurt a little.
Does this hurt?　　　Let me know if it hurts.
Now we're finished.　Now it's over. That's all.
Please press hard without massaging.
Please massage thoroughly.
Let me know if the place around the needle begins to hurt or look red.
Don't bathe today.
You can take a shower as long as your arm doesn't get wet.

☞　**2.　点滴に関する表現**

I'm going to give you an intravenous drip (injection).
It contains nutrients/ antibiotics.
It'll take about one hour to finish, so you'd better go to the toilet beforehand.
Please let us know if you feel hot.
Your IV is set to run at 70 drops per minute.

☞　**3.　指示の表現**

Unbutton your shirt for me, please.
Can you lift your right arm ?
Could you say "99" for me please?
Would you mind lying back on the bed?

語彙・表現: 感染症と予防接種

感染症関連用語

avian influenza	鳥インフルエンザ	acquired immunodeficiency syndrome[AIDS]	エイズ
swine influenza	豚(新型)インフルエンザ	human immunodeficiency virus [HIV]	HIVウイルス
polio	ポリオ、小児麻痺	sexually transmitted disease [STD]	性感染症
mumps	おたふく風邪	dengue fever	デング熱
malaria	マラリア	gastroenteritis	[急性感染性]胃腸炎
cholera	コレラ	West Nile fever	西ナイル熱
diphtheria	ジフテリア	Preventive Vaccination Law	予防接種法
rubella [German measles]	風疹	Global Program on AIDS [GPA]	エイズ対策特別計画
Japanese encephalitis	日本脳炎	Public Health Service Act [PHSA]	公衆衛生法(米)
chicken pox	水痘	measures for communicable disease control	伝染病対策
typhoid	腸チフス	surveillance system for tuberculosis and infectious diseases	結核・感染症サーベイランスシステム
rabies	狂犬病	quarantine	検疫[所、期間];隔離
parrot fever	オウム病		
the plague	ペスト		
pneumococcus	肺炎球菌		
yellow fever	黄熱病		
hepatitis A, B, C	A型・B型・C型肝炎		
severe acute respiratory syndrome[SARS]	重症急性呼吸器症候群		

予防接種や渡航歴に関する表現

When did you have a vaccination shot for measles?

What vaccinations have you had?

When was your last shot for it?

Have you had vaccinations [immunizations] for whooping cough?

Have you had any problems after the shot?

When did you last have a physical checkup?

Did they find anything wrong with you?

You'll have the next vaccination in about three weeks.

Have you ever traveled anywhere outside Japan?

Which countries did you go to, and how long did you stay there?

What was the purpose of your trip?

Was it a business trip or a pleasure trip?

Unit 7
Vital Signs

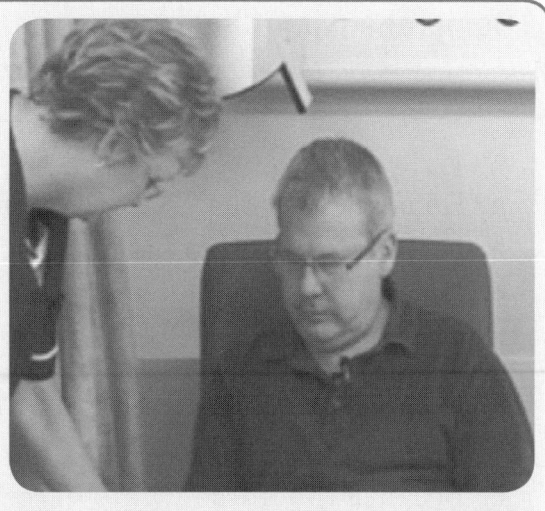

バイタルサインを測ることは、退院までの病棟での日課です。患者さんとの信頼関係を築く好機として大切にしましょう。

I Key Sentences

Check the sentences below, and read them aloud to memorize them.

1. I am going to take your temperature.
2. I just want to be sure about your condition.
3. Are you feeling warm enough?
4. We are looking forward to seeing your friends.
5. The doctor will be back tonight.

II Improve Your Communication Skills　　Play Both

Watch the bad and good dialogues, and answer the following questions.

1. the good dialogueではどのような点が改善されていたでしょうか。
2. 患者さんがどのように答えているか注意して書き出してみましょう。

III Comprehension Check

Watch the good dialogue and choose the most appropriate answer to each question on the DVD.

1. **Q:** [   ]
    a. He is going to the recovery room.
    b. He is going back to his house.
    c. He is going to come back to the hospital.

2. **Q:** [   ]
    a. Because the nurse wants to talk with him.
    b. Because the patient seems uneasy.
    c. Because the nurse wants to confirm the patient's physical condition.

3. **Q:** [   ]
    a. He is looking forward to going home.
    b. He isn't looking forward to anything special.
    c. He is looking forward to meeting the nurses again.

4. **Q:** [   ]
    a. Because he feels the nurses are very kind to him.
    b. Because he knows that he has recovered quite well.
    c. Because he likes nurses better than doctors.

IV Complete the Dialogue

Watch the good dialogue again and fill in the blanks.

(N: Nurse P: Patient)

N: Hello, Pete.

P: Hello.

N: I'm just going to take your (1)_____ if that's all right.

P: Oh, yes.

N: Just before you go home, I just want (2)_____ _____ _____ that it's OK. All right? Okeydoke. Good. OK, thank you very much. That's fine. Are you feeling all right?

P: Yes. I'm fine, thank you.

Unit 7   Vital Signs

N: (3)_____ _____ _____ going home.

P: I am indeed, yes.

N: OK, all right. We'll be back with you (4)_____ _____ _____.

P: OK, (5)_____ _____, thanks. Thanks.

V Substitution Practice

Replace the shaded expressions with those below and read them aloud.

1. Please relax and breathe out deeply .
   - breathe in deeply
   - hold your breath
   - lie down on the bed

2. Do you feel feverish ?
   - listless
   - chilly
   - cold
   - nauseous

3. What is your normal temperature ?
   - blood pressure
   - heart rate
   - respiratory rate

4. Don't open your mouth .
   - move
   - bend your knees
   - get nervous
   - close your eyes

VI Expand Your Vocabulary

From the box below, choose and write down the English words with the same meaning as the following Japanese words.

入院 _____   呼吸 _____

体温 _____   血圧 _____

体温計 _____   血圧計 _____

聴診器 _____   退院 _____

舌 _____   汗 _____

> stethoscope   temperature   tongue
> hospitalization   discharge   blood pressure
> sphygmomanometer   sweat   breath
> thermometer

VII Speaking Practice

1. the good dialogueを見て自分で練習してよく覚えましょう。
2. ペアになり役割を交代して練習しましょう。
3. 次は看護師Taylorさんの今日の予定です。Nurse Taylor is going to do を使って順序よく話してみましょう。

12 noon	Arrive at work
First thing	Check if there's a bed free for Mr. McDonald yet
2 p.m.	Give Mr. Carr a bedbath
3 p.m.	Accompany Dr. Patel on his ward-rounds
4 p.m.	Have a break!
6 p.m.	Do paperwork

Unit 7 　Vital Signs

いろいろな表現を覚えましょう

☞ 　体温、血圧などの表現

What is your usual blood pressure?
Please put your arm inside this white cuff.
Let me put this cuff on your arm.
Your blood pressure is 155 over 84.
You must keep the thermometer under your arm for three minutes.
Remove the thermometer when you hear the beeping sound.
Your temperature is 36.5°C (degrees centigrade) or 97.7°F (degrees Fahrenheit).
Please hold out your right hand.
Your pulse is 80 a minute.

体温・体重・身長の換算

```
換算式

温度:   カ氏           °F  = □℃×9/5+32
        セ氏           ℃   = (□°F−32)×5/9
重さ:   ポンド          lb. = □kg × 2.2
        キログラム      kg  = □lb. × 0.45
長さ:   フィート        ft. = □cm × 0.033
        センチメートル  cm  = □ft. × 30.5
        インチ          in. = □cm × 0.4
        センチメートル  cm  = □in. × 2.54
```

換算してみましょう
①カ氏98度(98°F) ②132ポンド(132 pounds) ③5フィート7インチ(5 feet 7 inches)をそれぞれセ氏、キログラム、センチメートルに換算してみましょう。

① カ氏 → セ氏:
98°F   ℃ = (□°F−32)×5/9
                  = (98−32)×5/9
                  = [   ]
98°F ≒ 36.7℃
Ninety-eight degrees Fahrenheit
≒ Thirty-six point seven degrees centigrade/Celsius

② ポンド → キログラム
132lb.   kg = □lb. × 0.45
                   = 132×0.45
                   = [   ]

③ フィート・インチ → センチメートル
5ft. 7in.   cm = (□ft. × 30.5)+(□in. × 2.54)
                   = (5×30.5)+(7×2.54)
                   = [   ]

Unit 8
Rehabilitation and Asking Questions

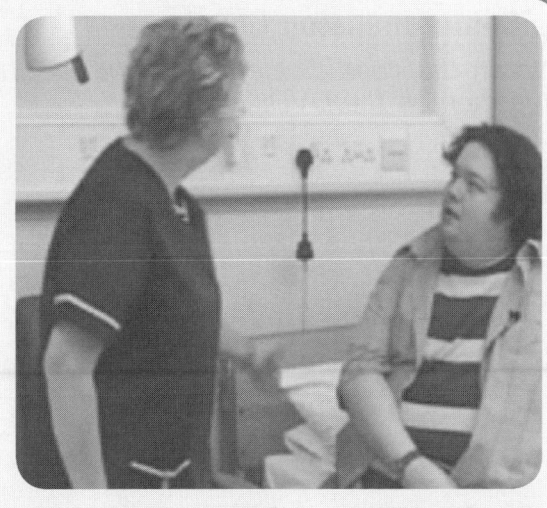

患者さんが転科する場合など、その理由を丁寧に説明し、環境変化への不安を取り除いてあげましょう。

I Key Sentences

Check the sentences below, and read them aloud to memorize them.

1. We're ready to take you to the rehabilitation unit.
2. They're going to help you get ready to go home.
3. They're really good at doing rehabilitation.
4. I'll miss you.
5. I'll go and organize a wheelchair.

II Improve Your Communication Skills　Play Both

Watch the bad and good dialogues, and answer the following questions.

1. the good dialogueではどのような点が改善されていましたか。
2. 患者さんはなぜ心を開いてリハビリテーション科への移動を受け入れていったと思いますか。

III Comprehension Check

Watch the good dialogue and choose the most appropriate answer to each question on the DVD.

1. **Q:** [   ]
   a. Home   b. To another hospital   c. To the rehabilitation unit

2. **Q:** [   ]
   a. She is standing beside him.
   b. She is sitting on the chair near the bed.
   c. She is sitting on the bed.

3. **Q:** [   ]
   a. Because rehabilitation is necessary.
   b. Because the patient hopes to go there.
   c. Because the nurses hope he will go there.

4. **Q:** [   ]
   a. She mentions the good skills of the experts there.
   b. She mentions the sudden change of his mood.
   c. She says that he wasn't a good patient in her unit.

IV Complete the Dialogue

Watch the good dialogue again and fill in the blanks.

(N: Nurse P: Patient)

N: Hi, Charles.

P: Hello.

N: All right? How are you feeling?

P: Yeah, I'm all right, thank you.

N: Good. Well, you know (1)_____ _____ now to take you over to the rehabilitation unit.

P: Mmm.

N: And you know that (2)_____ _____, there are people that are going to help you get ready to go home.

P: Mmm, OK.

N: (3)_____ _____, and they're really (4)_____ _____ _____ doing this, so don't...don't worry.

P: OK.

N: Right, and we'll be sorry that you're going and (5)_____ _____ _____, but I think that you'll get on (6)_____ _____ there.

P: Thank you (7)_____ _____ _____ _____.

N: I'll go and organize a wheelchair.

P: Yeah.

N: All right.

P: Thank you.

V Substitution Practice

Replace the shaded expressions with those below and read them aloud.

1. We're ready to take you to the rehabilitation unit.
   I'm ready
   I'm not ready
   She's ready
   The staff isn't ready

2. They are really good at doing rehabilitation.
   good at wrapping bandages
   good at calming down the patients
   poor at explaining their emotions

3. You'll get on really well at the rehabilitation unit.
   at the internal unit
   at the dermatology department
   in the nursing home
   in your workplace

45

4. I'll go and | organize a wheelchair | .
   organize your hospitalization
   organize your operation
   order a corset
   order a walker

VI Expand Your Vocabulary

From the box below, choose and write down the English words with the same meaning as the following Japanese words.

松葉杖 _____   皮膚科 _____

精神科 _____   職場 _____

老人ホーム _____   専門家 _____

紹介状 _____   コルセット _____

ギプス _____   感情 _____

crutch	emotion	dermatology department
cast	expert	psychiatry department
corset	nursing home	referral letter
workplace		

VII Speaking Practice

1. the good dialogueを見て自分で練習してよく覚えましょう。
2. ペアになり役割を交代して練習しましょう。
3. ナースが立ったまま患者さんと話す時と、患者さんと同じ目の高さで話す時をお互いに体験し、感想を述べてみましょう

Unit 8　Rehabilitation and Asking Questions

いろいろな表現を覚えましょう

☞ 1. 専門医（科）への紹介の表現

You need to see a heart/lung specialist.
I am going to refer you to a cancer specialist.
Let me refer you to another unit/hospital.
I'd be happy to write a referral letter.

☞ 2. リハビリテーション科での表現

You need to have some physical/occupational/speech therapy for your rehabilitation.
You need to come here for electrotherapy.
Please come to this center for cervical traction.
Please come here for massage on the knee twice a day.
I'm going to assess the mobility and strength of your arm.

☞ 3. 質問の種類と例

(1) Closed questions — to get a very specific or short piece of information
   How old are you?　　What tablets do you take?

(2) Open questions — to invite the patient to give a longer answer or tell a story
   Can you tell me what happened?　　How is the pain?
   What do your family think about this?

(3) Probing questions — to get more information about something that has already been said
   You said you felt frightened, what do you mean by 'frightened'?
   How often do you get the headaches?

Important Communication Skills in Nursing

グローバル化や、それに伴う感染症の問題でいろいろな国の患者さんが病院を訪れる機会が増加しています。医療コミュニケーションに関しては、人間としての共通な生物学的な部分、文化、歴史、風土などによって異なる部分、個人的な好みの問題もあり、現実の情報、知識、感情、意思の伝達表現は非常に微妙な点を含んでいます。ここでは主として欧米人とのコミュニケーションの特徴を説明しています。

Eye Contact
一般的に日本人はしっかり相手の目を見ることが少ないようですが、信頼され誠実な気持ちを伝えるには患者さんの目を見て話すことが大切です。

Listening and Checking
真剣に患者さんの気持ちを理解するように努力したり、また、あいづちを打つことはもちろん大切ですが、分からない場合は落ち着いて確かめ、必要なら看護行為につなげましょう。入浴方法や食事の献立など思いもよらない習慣の違いなどがあるものです。

Reflecting
患者さんの状況・環境などをよく考えてから話をするように。また自分の言動も慎重に顧みることが関係をスムーズにしてくれるでしょう。

Showing empathy
同情ではなく、患者さんに共感（I understand how you feel）を感じられるような感性を養い、それを日本人に対してより少し強めに表現しましょう。看護の重要な一部なので心理学上の知見にも興味・関心を持ちましょう。

Not using 'medical' words and Speaking clearly
患者さんには難しい医学用語は避け、分かりやすい言葉で話しましょう。また、英語を上手に話すことより、はっきりと話すことが大切です。'No' や 'I don't know' を曖昧にしておくと信頼を失うかもしれないので、特に注意しましょう。

Being kind
相手を尊重し、おせっかいな感じを与えないように気をつけましょう。

Body language
握手とか、手を振る向きとか、会話する時にお互いに不快を感じない距離とか、文化・年齢・性別による差があり非常に微妙です。注意深く観察して、時には相手に確かめた方がいいでしょう。また、日本人の身振り・手振りなどについて説明することもコミュニケーションの活性化に役立つでしょう。

Using cues and Asking questions
自分の方から話のきっかけを作ったり、積極的に質問をしたりして、異国にいる患者さんが話しやすいように心掛け、楽しくいい関係を作っていきましょう。

Negotiating
患者さん、医師、他の医療従事者との交渉では、習慣や文化の違いに注目し相手によく確かめ、感情的にならず辛抱強く交渉をまとめ、決まったら明確なフィードバックを忘れないようにしましょう。

Summarizing
重要事項の伝達のときなど、要領よくまとめ、時にはメモや図にして渡す方法もあります。そして、必ず確認する習慣を身に付けましょう。

Giving Information
正確な情報を丁寧に伝えましょう。英語での口頭説明が難しく複雑な場合など、説明書を準備しておくことも大切です。そして、選択可能な項目や内容などの補足説明などを忘れないようにしましょう。

Unit 9
Operation

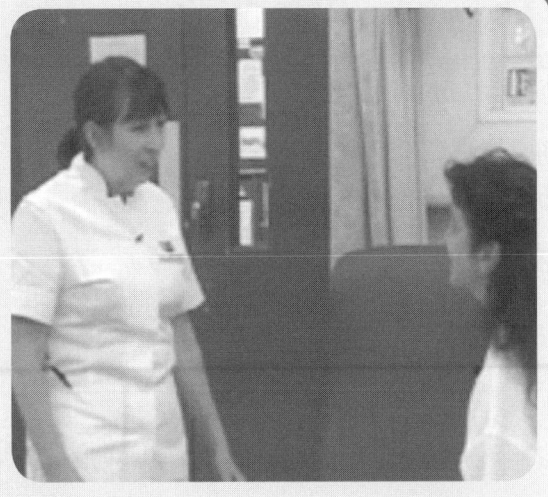

手術は医療者サイドにとっても重大事です。お互い連携してその前後の準備や指示を行い、患者さんへの再度の確認を忘れず、手術を成功させましょう。

I Key Sentences

Check the sentences below, and read them aloud to memorize them.

1. You are going to theater (the OR) today, aren't you?
2. You mustn't have anything to eat or drink.
3. The doctor explained last night.
4. We'll take you down to theater.
5. The operation begins at midday.

II Improve Your Communication Skills   Play Both

Watch the bad and good dialogues, and answer the following questions.

1. the good dialogueではどのような点が改善されていましたか。
2. 患者さんが不安感や安心感を抱いたりするのは、どのようなことが原因だと思いますか。

III Comprehension Check

Watch the good dialogue and choose the most appropriate answer to each question on the DVD.

1. **Q:** [   ]
   a. Not to eat anything   b. To sleep well   c. Not to eat or drink

2. **Q:** [   ]
   a. The previous lunchtime   b. The previous afternoon
   c. The previous night

3. **Q:** [   ]
   a. She has a fairly good impression of him.
   b. She has an unfavorable impression of him.
   c. She has an excellent impression of him.

4. **Q:** [   ]
   a. At midday   b. At once   c. In the middle of the night

IV Complete the Dialogue

Watch the good dialogue again and fill in the blanks.

(N: Nurse P: Patient)

N: Hello, Mary, how are you?

P: I'm fine, thank you.

N: That's good. You're going down (1)_____ _____ today, aren't you?

P: Yes.

N: And you have been told that you mustn't have anything (2)_____ _____ _____, haven't you?

P: The doctor (3)_____ _____ _____ last night. He seemed (4)_____ _____.

N: Yes, he's (5)_____ _____ _____. So somebody will come and (6)_____ _____ _____ to theater at about 12 o'clock

Unit 9 Operation

(7)_____.

P: Thank you.

N: OK? (8) _____ _____ _____.

V Substitution Practice

Replace the shaded expressions with those below and read them aloud.

1. You mustn't eat or drink anything .
   drink any alcohol
   smoke
   move your legs and feet
   sit up

2. You've been told that you must go to the recovery room .
   go to psychiatry first
   take off your shoes
   be careful

3. We will take you to the operation room soon.
   the cafeteria
   the treatment room
   the recovery room
   the delivery room

4. You'll be on a post-operative diet for several days.
   a liquid diet
   a diabetic diet
   a solid diet
   a low-salt diet

VI. Expand Your Vocabulary

From the box below, choose and write down the English words with the same meaning as the following Japanese words.

全身麻酔 _____ 局所麻酔 _____

消毒 _____ 痛み止め _____

同意書 _____ 手術控室 _____

回復室 _____ 普通食 _____

緩下剤 _____ 輸血 _____

```
painkiller         recovery room         general anesthesia
regular diet       pre-operative room    sterilization
transfusion        consent form          local anesthesia
laxative
```

VII. Speaking Practice

1. the good dialogueを見て自分で練習してよく覚えましょう。
2. ペアになり、役割を交代して練習しましょう。
3. ペアになり、軽い胃の内視鏡手術の患者さんに必要な術前の注意をしてみましょう。

いろいろな表現を覚えましょう

☞ **1. 手術に関する表現**

Have you ever had surgery?

Please take out your dentures or contact lenses, and take off your rings.

Do you have any allergies to anesthesia and other medication?

You'll be given general/local anesthesia.

You'll feel a bit drowsy afterwards, but that's all.

The whole team are very good so you're in safe hands.

The surgery will be over before you know it.

You may need a blood transfusion.
You can walk on the day after the operation.
Your surgery was successful.
You had a hard time, but you've made it.
You can go back to your room in 30 minutes or so.
I am going to give you mouthwash.
Please let us know when you passed gas.

2. 同意書に関する表現

This is the consent form for your operation.
If you have any questions, the doctor will explain in detail.
Please take time to read this consent form carefully, and sign here.
Do you have anyone who can sign it for you?

3. 痛みに関する表現

Where does it hurt?
What kind of pain is it?
Is it painful to touch?
Tell me about the pain in your back, please.
Just let me know right away if it starts to hurt.
I have a pain around my abdomen.
It's a severe pain (a slight pain, a dull pain, a sharp pain,
a throbbing pain, a constant pain, an intermittent pain,
a localized pain, a widespread pain).
When did the pain start?   Yesterday./ Two hours ago.

健康に関することわざ

健康については古来からさまざまな「ことわざ」が語り継がれています。英語と日本語のことわざを比べてみましょう。

Care killed a cat. / Worry often causes illness.	心配は身の毒
Habit (Custom) is a second nature.	習慣は第二の天性
Hunger is the best sauce.	空腹にまずいものなし
Prevention is better than cure.	予防は治療に勝る
Sound mind in a sound body.	健全な精神は健全な身体に宿る
Tongue ever turns to the aching tooth.	心配事は心から離れない
You are what you eat.	命は食にあり
Starve a fever, feed a cold.	熱には食べず、風邪には食べよ
Everything starts with a cold.	風邪は万病の元
An apple a day keeps the doctor away.	1日1個のリンゴで医者いらず
Do all things in moderation.	過ぎたるは及ばざるがごとし
One ailment will make you more attentive to your health.	一病息災
A good medicine tastes bitter.	良薬は口に苦し
Time is a great healer.	時は偉大な治療者
Good wine engenders good blood.	酒は百薬の長

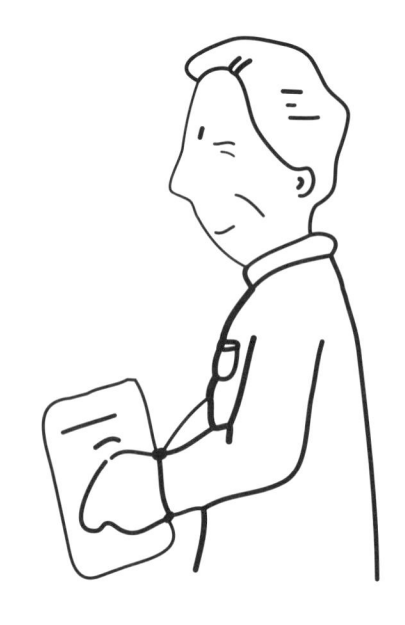

Unit 10
Positioning the Patient and Giving Instructions

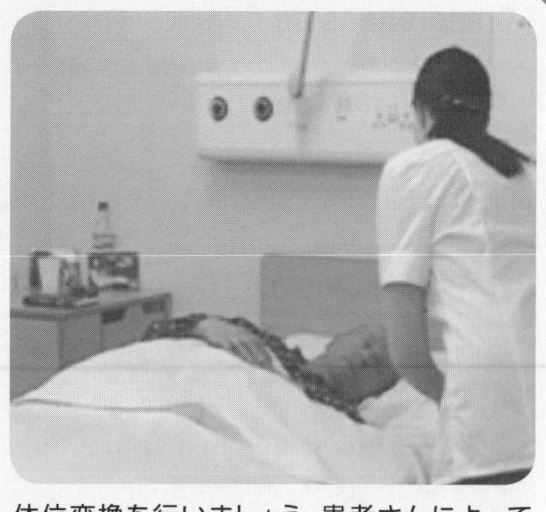

患者さんの微妙な心身の反応をよく把握し、体位変換を行いましょう。患者さんによっては自力で出来る部分もあるかもしれません。

I Key Sentences

Check the sentences below, and read them aloud to memorize them.

1. Are you all right like this?
2. We are going to move you backward.
3. I could do with a cushion.
4. Lie down on the bed slowly.
5. Does that feel worse?

II Improve Your Communication Skills　　Play Both

Watch the bad and good dialogues, and answer the following questions.

1. the good dialogueではどのような点が改善されていましたか。
2. 患者さんの体位や身体を動かす場合、どのような点に関して注意が必要でしょうか。

III Comprehension Check

Watch the good dialogue and choose the most appropriate answer to each question on the DVD.

1. **Q:** [   ]
   a. Because he points to the pillows.
   b. Because he seems uncomfortable.
   c. Because she has to check the pillow cases.

2. **Q:** [   ]
   a. She finds it on the side of his bed.
   b. She finds it has just fallen onto the chair.
   c. She finds it on the floor.

3. **Q:** [   ]
   a. He suggests that she put the pillow under his head.
   b. He suggests that she put the pillow on the chair.
   c. He suggests that she put the pillow at the bottom of his bed.

4. **Q:** [   ]
   a. She first lets him get out of bed.
   b. She first takes another pillow from his head.
   c. She first moves him forward.

IV Complete the Dialogue

Watch the good dialogue again and fill in the blanks.

(N: Nurse P: Patient)

N: Oh, Rob, that (1)_____ _____ very comfortable. You all right (2)_____ _____?

P: I could do (3)_____ _____ _____ _____, please.

N: OK, that's fine. Right, I'm gonna (4)_____ _____ _____.

P: OK.

N: (5)_____ _____ _____?

P: Yes, fine, thank you.

N: OK. And then if you…you're going to (6)_____ _____ _____.

Is that all right? Does that feel (7)_____?

P: (8)_____ _____, _____.

N: Yeah. OK, I'll see you later.

V Substitution Practice

Replace the shaded expressions with those below and read them aloud.

1. | Are you all right | like this?
   | Are you satisfied with the room |
   | Are you satisfied with your diet |
   | Do you want your coffee |

2. I am going to | move you | to the treatment room.
   | take him |
   | carry her |
   | walk them |

3. Please lie | down |.
   | down on your stomach |
   | on your back |
   | on your right side |

4. I am going to change | your position | now.
   | your sheet and pillow cases |
   | your bandage |
   | your hospital gown |
   | the air in your room |

VI Expand Your Vocabulary

From the box below, choose and write down the English words with the same meaning as the following Japanese words.

仰臥位 _____　　寝たきりの _____

床ずれ（じょくそう）_____　（枕を）ふくらます _____

（シーツなどを）直す _____　移動 _____

床上安静 _____　支える _____

転倒 _____　　座位 _____

```
bed rest          straighten        sitting position
fluff             transfer          bedsore
support           bedridden         supine position
fall
```

VII Speaking Practice

1. 動画を見て自分で練習してよく覚えましょう。
2. ペアになり、役割を交代して練習しましょう。
3. 高齢の女性患者さんにまずベッドで寝てもらい、それから枕を直すために起き上がってもらう場面の会話をペアで行ってみましょう。

Unit 10　Positioning the Patient and Giving Instructions

いろいろな表現を覚えましょう

☞ **1. 体位交換などの指示表現**

Please turn over.　　　　　Turn to the left.
Would you sit up?　　　　Sit on the bed, please.
Please roll over onto your back.
Please stretch out your legs.
Could you please put your feet up?
Please hold my hand.

☞ **2. その他の体位に関する表現**

I had the patient sit on the edge of the bed.
I'll raise the bed to place you in a supine position.
I'll support your back so that you can stand up without falling.
In order to prevent bedsores, we have to change the patient's position every two hours.

☞ **3. 患者さんを励ましながら動かす表現**

Try and walk to the end of the bed.
Let's see if you can walk without the stick (cane).
Well done!
Good for you!
A bit more!

Pain Scale

Pain		ADL
Intolerable (我慢できない激痛)	10	Completely interferes with ADL
Considerable (かなりの激痛)	8	Greatly interferes with ADL
Oppressive (苦しみを伴う痛み)	6	Partially interferes with ADL
Tolerable (我慢できる痛み)	4	Somewhat interferes with ADL
Minor discomfort (気にならない程度の痛み)	2	Mildly interferes with ADL
None (痛みなし)	0	Does not interferes with ADL

***Activities of Daily Living (ADL)**
Such as: sleeping, eating, mood, walking, enjoyment of life relationships

Unit 11
Medication

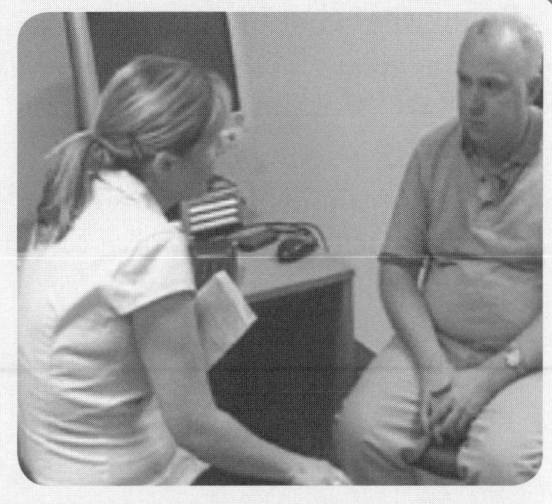

投薬には複雑で正確な説明を要します。患者さんの声の調子にも注意して、分かりやすい表現や確認の仕方を考えましょう。

I Key Sentences

Check the sentences below, and read them aloud to memorize them.

1. From our assessment, you have a clinical depression.
2. Here's a prescription for you.
3. These tablets take two to three weeks to really work.
4. It's best to take these tablets with breakfast.
5. I'll take these tablets with breakfast.

II Improve Your Communication Skills — Play Both

Watch the bad and good dialogues, and answer the following questions.

1. the good dialogueではどのような点が改善されていたでしょうか。
2. 患者さんが精神疾患を患っていたり、子供だったり、眼や耳が不自由なときはどのように薬の飲み方を伝え、確認するか、書き出してみましょう。

III Comprehension Check

Watch the good dialogue and choose the most appropriate answer to each question on the DVD.

1. **Q:** [   ]
   a. Medication will help him.　　b. Relaxation is all that he needs.
   c. The patient doesn't have to come again.

2. **Q:** [   ]
   a. Two weeks　　　　b. Two to three weeks　　　c. Three months

3. **Q:** [   ]
   a. Every other day　　b. Once in five days　　　c. Every day

4. **Q:** [   ]
   a. Low and sad mood　　　　b. Headaches and tiredness
   c. Headaches and sickness

IV Complete the Dialogue

Watch the good dialogue again and fill in the blanks.

(N: Nurse P: Patient)

N: OK, so (1)_____ _____ _____, you have a clinical depression.

P: Yeah.

N: But (2)_____ _____ _____ is medication does help…

P: OK.

N: …with depressions like this, and in time, you will be feeling a lot better.

P: Mm-hmm.

N: Now, (3)_____ _____ _____ _____ here for you. Can I explain just a little about (4)_____ _____?

P: Yeah, sure.

N: What they'd seem to work on is (5)_____ _____ _____

_____ _____ to help level things out so you're more on an even keel and lift your mood a little.

P: OK.

N: You should feel more relaxed.

P: Relaxed. Yeah, OK.

N: But they take two to three weeks to really kick in and (6)_____.

P: OK.

N: You'll need to take them every day.

P: Yeah.

N: (7)_____ _____ _____ _____ with breakfast.

P: With breakfast, yeah.

N: And, um, there are a few side effects, er, that some people get –

(8)_____ _____ _____.

P: Right.

N: Headaches, sickness. If...but if you take the time to read the leaflet through, that comes with the tablets in the box...

P: OK.

N: ...it'll explain very well (9)_____ _____ _____ _____ _____.

P: OK.

N: But any problems at all, do come back, or give me a phone call at the surgery.

P: OK. Thank you, nurse.

N: Do you have (10)_____ _____?

P: No.

N: No? You sure now?

P: Yeah.

N: OK.

P: OK, thank you.

V Substitution Practice

Replace the shaded expressions with those below and read them aloud.

1. You'll be more on an even keel .
   - more relaxed
   - more refreshed
   - better informed

2. You'll need to take five pills four times a day .
   - twice a day
   - every eight hours

3. You should take this powdered medicine before meals .
   - with your meals
   - at bedtime
   - between meals

4. Please give us a phone call if you have any problems .
   - if your symptoms do not improve
   - if your symptoms become worse
   - if you notice any side effects

VI Expand Your Vocabulary

From the box below, choose and write down the English words with the same meaning as the following Japanese words.

化学物質 _____   ちらし _____

処方箋 _____   高揚させる _____

吐き気 _____   症例、事例 _____

(薬が)効く _____ 重篤な _____

粉薬 _____   安定させる _____

```
lift              work          powdered medicine
prescription      serious       chemical
level out         case          sickness
leaflet
```

Unit 11　Medication

VII Speaking Practice

1. the good dialogueを見て自分で練習してよく覚えましょう。
2. ペアになり、役割を交代して練習しましょう。
3. 患者さんに laxative, painkiller, antidepressantなどを与える会話をペアで行ってみましょう。

いろいろな表現を覚えましょう

☞ 1. 投薬などに関する表現

This is a prescription for your medication.
Hand over the prescription at the counter of the pharmacy.
Pay at the cashier's window, and then pick up your medication at the pharmacy.
Do you have any drug allergies?
This medicine is good for your stomachache.
You have two kinds of medicine.
Take this capsule within 30 minutes after each meal.
Take one tablet at a time when you have pain.
Take these pills twice a day for four weeks.
You can stop taking this cold medicine if you get better.
Please stop using this ointment if you feel itchy.
Please put in eye drops.
Please give this cough syrup to your baby.
Please dissolve this tablet under your tongue.
The medication will start working in a minute or two.
This will make you sleepy, so don't drive or operate machinery.

☞ 2. 薬の種類

compress, fever reducer, mouthwash, antipruritic, antisuppuration, laxative, antidiarrhetic, antibiotics, sleeping pills, stomach medicine, vitamin pills

資料　　　　語彙：疾病と創傷（１）

BONE, MUSCLE, JOINT　骨,筋,関節

fracture (fx)	骨折
sprain	ねんざ

BRAIN AND NERVOUS SYSTEM　脳・神経系

stroke	脳卒中
brain tumor	脳腫瘍
dementia	認知症
Alzheimer's disease	アルツハイマー病
Parkinson's disease	パーキンソン病

MENTAL ILLNESS　精神疾患

mania	躁病
depression	うつ病
insomnia	不眠症
neurosis	ノイローゼ, 神経症
eating disorder	摂食障害

RESPIRATORY SYSTEM　呼吸器系

pneumonia	肺炎
lung cancer	肺がん
tuberculosis (TB)	結核
bronchitis	気管支炎

CIRCULATORY SYSTEM　循環器系

heart disease	心臓病
heart attack	心臓発作
heart failure	心不全

DIGESTIVE SYSTEM　消化器系

hepatitis	肝炎
liver cirrhosis	肝硬変
liver cancer; hepatic cancer	肝臓がん
colon cancer	大腸がん
appendicitis	虫垂炎(盲腸炎)
food poisoning	食中毒

KIDNEY AND URINARY SYSTEM　腎・泌尿器系

cystitis	膀胱炎
kidney failure	腎不全

BLOOD AND IMMUNE SYSTEM　血液・免疫系

anemia	貧血
leukemia	白血病

接頭辞 (prefix)

a-	（無）	anemia 貧血	apnea 無呼吸
in-	（不）	insomnia 不眠症	inability 無能
hyper-	（過剰）	hypertension 高血圧	hypermetabolism 代謝亢進
hypo-	（過少）	hypotension 低血圧	hypothermia 低体温症
post-	（後の）	postnatal 生後の	postoperative 術後の
pre-	（前の）	prenatal 出生前の	premedication 前投薬
psych(o)	（精神）	psychiatry 精神医学	psychotherapy 精神・心理療法

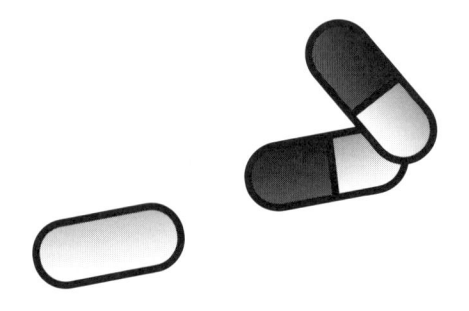

Unit 12
Discharge and Goodbye

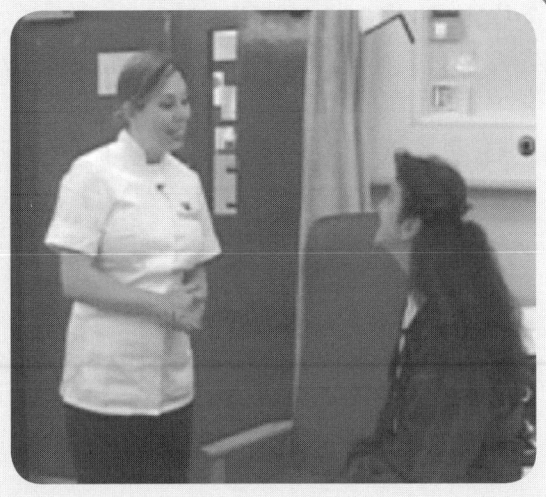

終わり良ければ、すべてよし——退院患者さんを気持ちよく送り出すにはどのようにしたらよいか考えましょう。

I Key Sentences

Check the sentences below, and read them aloud to memorize them.

1. I'm waiting for a lift (ride).
2. You do look much better.
3. It's been quite a busy week.
4. Did you have trouble walking?
5. I hope you have a safe journey (trip) home.

II Improve Your Communication Skills   Play Both

Watch the bad and good dialogues, and answer the following questions.

1. the good dialogueではどのようなに改善されていたでしょうか。
2. 外来患者と入院患者に対する別れのあいさつにはどのような違いがあるか考えましょう。

III Comprehension Check

Watch the good dialogue and choose the most appropriate answer to each question on the DVD.

1. **Q:** [   ]
   a. The nurse
   b. An elevator
   c. Someone to take her home in the car

2. **Q:** [   ]
   a. Because the nurse wants to apologize to her.
   b. Because the nurse has a chance to say goodbye to her.
   c. Because the patient looks much better.

3. **Q:** [   ]
   a. The nurses are very busy at night.
   b. Her operation didn't go so well.
   c. The hospital is noisy at night.

4. **Q:** [   ]
   a. Because the patient had a bit of trouble sleeping.
   b. Because the nurse couldn't say goodbye before.
   c. Because the nurse didn't take good care of her.

IV Complete the Dialogue

Watch the good dialogue again and fill in the blanks.

(N: Nurse P: Patient)

N: Mary!

P: Oh, hello.

N: Hello. You're still here.

P: Yes, I'm waiting for (1)_____ _____.

N: Oh, well, this is good because I have a chance to (2)_____ _____ to you.

P: Oh, thank you.

N: It's been very nice to meet you.

Unit 12   Discharge and Goodbye

P: And you too.

N: And I hear your operation went very well.

P: Very well.

N: You (3)_____ _____ _____ _____.

P: Thank you.

N: So has everything been all right here for you?

P: Yes, but it has been (4)_____ _____ _____.

N: Mmm, it can be. It's been quite a busy week this week. Did you have trouble sleeping?

P: A little.

N: A little bit. (5)_____ _____ _____ _____ that.

P: That's all right. I understand.

N: Oh, thank you for that. Well, I hope you have (6)_____ _____ _____ _____.

P: Thank you.

N: Are you waiting for somebody?

P: Yes, I am.

N: Lovely. OK. I'll (7)_____ _____ _____ _____. Bye-bye.

P: Thank you very much.

N: Bye-bye

P: Bye-bye.

V Substitution Practice

Replace the shaded expressions with those below and read them aloud.

1. I have a chance to say goodbye to my patient .
   - to meet you again
   - to speak about rehabilitation
   - to recover my appetite

2. I am sorry about that .
   - this result
   - the careless mistakes

3. Did you have trouble sleeping ?
   - trouble hearing
   - trouble swallowing
   - trouble with your memory

4. I hope you have a safe journey home .
   - have a nice trip home
   - have a wonderful vacation in Karuizawa
   - had a good stay in this hospital

VI Expand Your Vocabulary

From the box below, choose and write down the English words with the same meaning as the following Japanese words.

帰宅の旅 _____   機会 _____

記憶 _____   食欲 _____

予約 _____   ホームヘルパー _____

休息する _____   飲み込む _____

指示する _____   安全な _____

```
rest            appointment        appetite
chance          journey home       swallow
safe            home-care aide     instruct
memory
```

Unit 12　Discharge and Goodbye

VII Speaking Practice

1. the good dialogueを見て自分で練習してよく覚えましょう。
2. ペアになり、役割を交代して練習しましょう。
3. ペアになり、退院したくなさそうな患者さんと看護師の会話を行ってみましょう。

いろいろな表現を覚えましょう

☞ **1. 退院の時の表現**

You can leave the hospital on May 10.
Congratulations on leaving the hospital.
We hope you get much better after your discharge.
Is someone coming to pick you up?
Please rest if you feel weak.
Please take your medication as instructed.

☞ **2. 退院後に関して**

Is there anyone who can help you prepare meals?
Please visit the hospital for a regular checkup.
Did you make an appointment for the next checkup?
Be sure to keep your follow-up appointment.
We have referred you to the rehabilitation facilities.
Do you need a home-care aide?

資料　　　語彙: 疾病と創傷（2）

ENDOCRINE SYSTEM　内分泌系
diabetes	糖尿病

WOMEN'S DISEASES
breast cancer	乳がん
menopausal disorder	更年期障害

EAR, NOSE, THROAT AND EYE　目,鼻,咽喉,眼
tonsillitis	扁桃炎
cataract (cat.)	白内障
blindness	失明

SKIN　皮膚
skin cancer	皮膚がん
burn	やけど, 熱傷
wart	いぼ

CHILDREN'S DISEASES　小児疾患
chickenpox	水痘
Down's syndrome	ダウン症
measles	はしか

DENTISTRY　歯科
decayed tooth	虫歯

WOUNDS　傷害
cut	切り傷
bump; lump	こぶ, たんこぶ

RELATED TERMS　関連用語
complication	合併症
acute disease	急性疾患
chronic disease	慢性疾患
benign	良性の
malignant	悪性の
innate; congenital; hereditary; inherited	先天性の
acquired	後天性の
malnutrition	栄養失調（症）

接尾辞 (suffix)

-ache　（痛）	headache 頭痛	stomachache 胃痛	toothache 歯痛
-itis　（炎症）	arthritis 関節炎	hepatitis 肝炎	nephritis 腎炎
-oma　（腫）	hematoma 血腫	myoma 筋腫	carcinoma がん

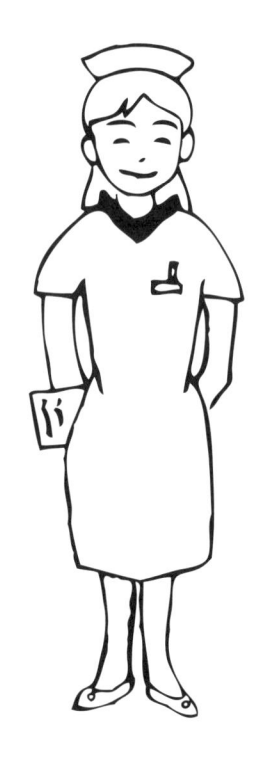

Unit 13
Negotiation Management

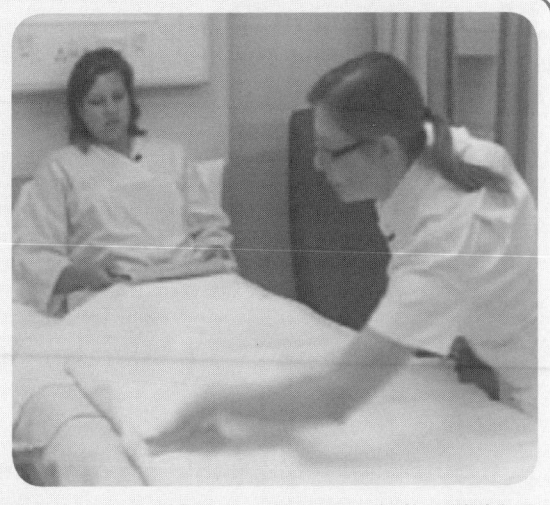

患者さんと医師や他のスタッフとの調整役をすることも仕事の一部です。自分の責任の域を守り、冷静で誠意ある表現を心掛けましょう。

I Key Sentences

Check the sentences below, and read them aloud to memorize them.

1. I hear you wanted a urinal.
2. I'm still in pain.
3. Can I talk to a head nurse?
4. I can see you look well.
5. I'll go and get the doctor for you.

II Improve Your Communication Skills **Play Both**

Watch the bad and good dialogues, and answer the following questions.

1. the good dialogueではどのような点が改善されていたでしょうか。
2. この看護師は患者さんの訴えと医師との間で、どのような対処法が考えられるか挙げてみましょう。

III Comprehension Check

Watch the good dialogue and choose the most appropriate answer to each question on the DVD.

1. **Q:** [   ]
   a. Her test results
   b. A blanket and her test results
   c. A blanket

2. **Q:** [   ]
   a. She is sleeping.   b. She is reading a newspaper.   c. She is crying.

3. **Q:** [   ]
   a. She still feels cold.   b. She is still depressed.
   c. She is still in pain.

4. **Q:** [   ]
   a. The nurse repeats that the test results are good.
   b. The nurse says that the doctor is pleased with her test results.
   c. The nurse decides to go and fetch the doctor for her.

IV Complete the Dialogue

Watch the good dialogue again and fill in the blanks.

(N: Nurse P: Patient)

N: Hello, Anna.

P: Hi.

N: I hear (1)_____ _____ _____ _____.

P: Yes, please.

N: Let me put this on for you.

P: (2)_____ _____ _____ to you about my test results?

N: Yes, if you like.

P: I'm really (3)_____ _____ about them because I'm (4)_____

_____ _____. Can I talk to a doctor?

N: Yes, I heard (5)_____ _____ were good. The doctor (6)_____ _____.

P: Yes, but I'm still in pain, so I'm not happy about it.

N: I can see you look very worried.

P: Yeah.

N: I'll go and (7)_____ _____ _____ for you.

P: (8)_____ _____ be good, yeah.

N: (9)_____ _____ able to explain. OK.

V Substitution Practice

Replace the shaded expressions with those below and read them aloud.

1. I hear you wanted   a blanket   .
   - a glass of water
   - a hot compress
   - a bedpan
   - nail clippers

2. We were pleased   with your test results   .
   - with the treatment
   - with your health condition
   - with your good response

3. Can I talk to   a doctor about my test results   ?
   - a doctor about my pain
   - a doctor about my worries
   - you about my family
   - you about my fear of an operation

4. I'll go and get the doctor for you.
　　　　　　 get the technician
　　　　　　 arrange the schedule
　　　　　　 fetch your friend

VI Expand Your Vocabulary

From the box below, choose and write down the English words with the same meaning as the following Japanese words.

調整する _____　　痛み止め _____

副作用 _____　　温湿布 _____

和らげる _____　　爪切り _____

毛布 _____　　連れてくる _____

（病床用）便器 _____　　反応 _____

```
painkiller          blanket         relieve
nail clippers       bedpan          arrange
hot compress        fetch           response
side effect
```

VII Speaking Practice

1. the good dialogueを見て自分で練習してよく覚えましょう。
2. ペアになり、役割を交代して練習しましょう。
3. 次のような課題をグループで解決しましょう。また、その話し合いの過程は患者さんとの話し合いでも変わらないか考えてみましょう。

　　Imagine the hospital has been given a gift of 10 million yen. You have 20 minutes to decide how the money is spent. If you do not decide, the money will be lost! You cannot ask anyone for help—you must decide yourself.

Unit 13　Negotiation　Management

いろいろな表現を覚えましょう

☞ **1.　患者さんの訴え（主訴）などを聞く表現**

Tell me why you came today.
How can I help you today?　　What can I do for you today?
Can you tell me about your problem?
What kind of concerns/difficulties/worries are you having?
How many days have you had the pain?
Do you have any other signs or symptoms?
What do you think is causing constipation?
How long does each stomachache last?
When do you usually get short of breath?
Does the dizziness come repeatedly or at regular intervals?
Does the toothache come on suddenly or gradually?
In what situations do you have a rapid heart rate?

☞ **2.　確認するための表現**

I beg your pardon?　　Pardon me?
Could you please say it again?　　Could you repeat that, please?
I'm sorry, I couldn't hear you.
What did you say?
Could you speak more slowly and clearly?
Tell me what you mean by saying you're anxious?
Could you write it on this paper?

☞ **3.　患者さんの発言を促す表現**

Please go on.
And what else?　Anything else?
Tell me more about the problems with your nose, please.
Give me a phone call later, please.

Tips for Nursing Communication

What would you say to a patient who told you to "go away" when you were trying to help?

This is about understanding how patients may feel or behave when they are ill. It is also about explaining the nurse role—why he or she needs to do the action. It is also about the nurse not feeling hurt.

What is negotiating?

It is about sharing decisions, and two people reaching an agreement. Sometimes it is about solving a problem when the nurse and the patient want different things.

What is counseling?

It is helping a patient to find his or her own answers. Skills include asking questions, listening, not judging, not suggesting answers and acknowledging emotion. It is about what the *patient* thinks. It is not about what the *nurse* thinks!

What things are important when breaking bad news?

It is important to be honest with patients. Tell the truth. Do not hide the news. If you do not know the answer to a question, say that you do not know. "I cannot say exactly because every patient is different but many patients with your illness live for over five years." It is important to allow the patient to talk by saying "Do you have any questions?", "You can ask me anything", "Tell me how you are feeling", etc.

How might nurses feel while they work with patients who are dying?

Nurses can feel sad. They can feel that they did not do enough. They can be unhappy because a person in their family also has a fatal illness. They may cry. It is important to tell the nurses that this is normal and OK. Nurses can talk to each other, and to their seniors.

Unit 14
Consultation (Pregnancy)

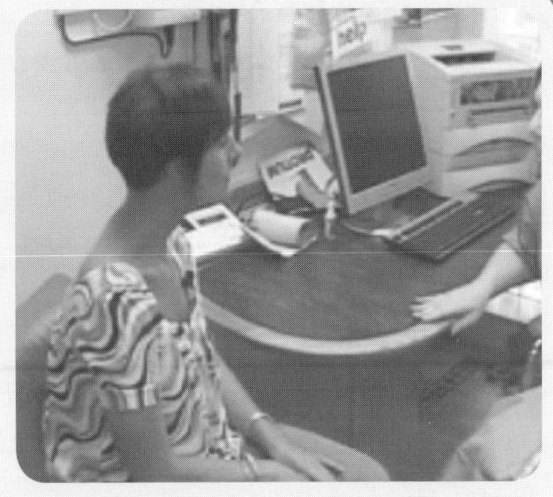

診断結果の説明や予後の方針を協議する際に、話しながら患者さんの希望や意思を引き出し、患者さん自身が決定するように導くプロセスを学びましょう。

Key Sentences

Check the sentences below, and read them aloud to memorize them.

1. I can confirm that you are pregnant.
2. I wasn't planning on having any more children.
3. It might be a good idea to surprise him.
4. Take time to think about it.
5. I'm here to listen and answer your questions.

Improve Your Communication Skills — Play Both

Watch the bad and good dialogues, and answer the following questions.

1. the good dialogueではどのような点が改善されていたでしょうか。
2. この患者さんのケースが難しいのは、なぜだと思いますか。

III Comprehension Check DVD CD 28 **Comprehension Check**

Watch the good dialogue and choose the most appropriate answer to each question on the DVD.

1. **Q:** [   ]
   a. She is pleased with the good news.   b. She is shocked.
   c. She doesn't know how to react.

2. **Q:** [   ]
   a. Having more than two children
   b. Speaking to her husband about the pregnancy
   c. Bringing her husband to the hospital

3. **Q:** [   ]
   a. No one   b. The nurse   c. The patient

4. **Q:** [   ]
   a. The nurse advises her to take a little time to decide about it herself.
   b. The nurse advises her not to tell her husband about it.
   c. The nurse advises her to keep it secret from her husband for a while.

IV Complete the Dialogue WEB動画 DVD CD 29 **Good Dialogue**

Watch the good dialogue again and fill in the blanks.

(N: Nurse P: Patient)

N: Well, Kate, I have the result of your test, and I can confirm that

(1)_____ _____ _____.

P: OK. Oh, it's a bit of a shock.

N: How are you feeling right now?

P: Um, slightly worried, (2)_____. Yeah, (3)_____ _____

planning on having any more children. So….

N: A surprise?

P: Yeah.

N: Yeah. So (4)_____ _____ _____ you're most worried

about?

Unit 14 Consultation (Pregnancy)

P: (5)_____ _____ _____ _____. You know, we already have two children, and weren't planning on having any more.

N: OK. Sounds like it might be (6)_____ _____ _____ to speak to him.

P: Yeah.

N: Yeah. Would you like to speak to your husband before we talk any more?

P: Yeah, I think I need to speak to him first, yes.

N: Would you like to (7)_____ _____ in with you?

P: Yeah, I think that would probably be helpful, once I've spoken to him, yes.

N: OK. Perhaps then you should speak to him this evening, take a little time, think about (8)_____ _____ _____.

P: OK.

N: And then come back and see me.

P: OK, yeah, that'll be good.

N: I'm...I'm here to listen and to answer your questions.

P: OK, thank you.

N: Whatever (9)_____ _____. OK?

P: OK. Thanks.

N: OK. You all right?

P: Yeah.

N: OK.

V Substitution Practice

Replace the shaded expressions with those below and read them aloud.

1. I can confirm that you are pregnant.
   your pregnancy test is positive/negative
   your baby is growing well
   your baby is in the breech/head down position

2. I wasn't planning on having more children.
   having a vaginal delivery
   a Cesarean delivery
   bottle feeding

3. Would you like to bring him in with you?
   see your baby now
   have maternity leave
   breast-feed your baby

4. I'm here to answer your questions.
   to explain childbirth methods
   to recommend the Lamaze technique of controlled breathing
   to measure your abdominal circumference

VI Expand Your Vocabulary

From the box below, choose and write down the English words with the same meaning as the following Japanese words.

母乳をやる _____   出産休暇 _____

未熟児 _____   腹囲 _____

双子 _____   息む _____

帝王切開による出産 _____   流産する _____

つわり _____   更年期障害 _____

```
breast-feed      morning sickness           Cesarean delivery
miscarry         premature baby             maternity leave
push             abdominal circumference    menopausal disorder
twins
```

Unit 14 Consultation (Pregnancy)

VII Speaking Practice

1. the good dialogueをペアになり、役割を交代して練習しましょう。
2. ペアになり、次のようなケースのカウンセリングではどのような質問をしたらいいか考え、実際に行ってみましょう。
   Imagine that a female patient is worried about her marriage. Her husband is always angry. She cannot sleep.

いろいろな表現を覚えましょう

☞ **1. 妊娠に関する表現**

When was the first day of your last menstrual period?
Do you have vomiting?
Do you have loss of appetite?
Do you have lower back pain?
Do you have swelling?
Congratulations! You must be pregnant.
Please get onto the table and put your feet in the supports.
Your due date is September 20.
Have you felt your baby moving?
Let's check the development of the fetus by ultrasound.

☞ **2. 分娩に関する表現**

Have you had any miscarriages or abortions?
Was your delivery normal?
Was your delivery a forceps delivery or vacuum extraction?
How long was your labor with the first child?
How far apart are your contractions?
Is it all right if we give you a drug to induce labor?
Has your water broken?
Please come to the delivery room with your wife during the birth.
Please try to comfort your baby.

Has your baby had any convulsive seizures?
Please hold your child so I can examine him.

👉 3. ウイメンズヘルスに関する表現

How long are your menstrual cycles?
Do you always have cramps before your period?
How often do you do breast self-examination?
What are you doing to prevent osteoporosis?
How old were you when you reached menopause?

資料　　　語彙：看護・医療用品

aspirator	吸引器	medication/IV cart	与薬・点滴カート
bed-pan	指し込み便器	monitor	監視装置
blood pressure gauge; sphygmomanometer	血圧計	naso-gastric tube	経鼻胃管
compressed air outlet	圧縮空気指し込みプラグ	oxygen tank	酸素タンク
crutch/crutches	松葉杖	respirator	人工呼吸装置
cuff	カフ(血圧計の加圧帯)	splint	副木
defibrillator	除細動器	steam inhaler	蒸気吸入器
drain tube	排水チューブ	stethoscope	聴診器
enema	浣腸(器)	stretcher	担架
gastric/stomach tube	胃管	tourniquet	止血帯, 圧迫帯
height scale	身長計	treatment table	処置台
infectious waste bin	危険物廃棄ボックス	urine bottle	採尿器、しびん
inhaler	吸入器	ventilator	人口呼吸器
intravenous injection (IV) pole	点滴用ポール	walker (with brakes)	歩行器(ブレーキ付き)
irrigator	洗浄器, イリガトール	wheelchair (WC)	車椅子
medical supplies	処置用品(具)	weight scale	体重計

Unit 15
Consultation (Cancer)

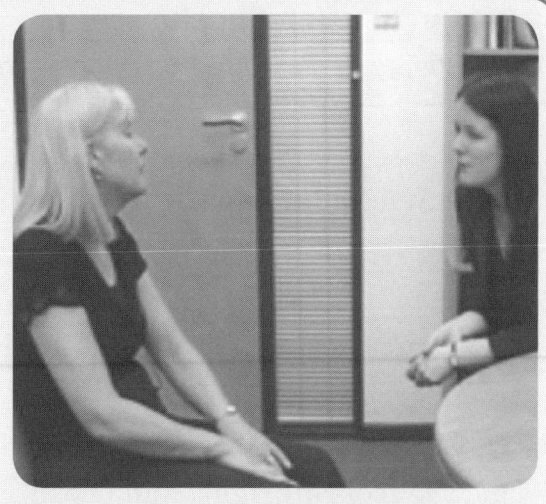

難しい病気の場合など、時間をかけて、患者さんの気持ちを尊重して落ち着かせ、受け入れ、相談にのる会話の進め方を学びましょう。

I Key Sentences

Check the sentences below, and read them aloud to memorize them.

1. Did he tell you your diagnosis?
2. It's a bit of a shock.
3. How have you been feeling?
4. It's natural to feel that way.
5. We can talk in more detail about what's happening.
6. We can tackle each of those in turn.

II Improve Your Communication Skills　WEB動画　DVD　Play Both

Watch the bad and good dialogues, and answer the following questions.

1. the good dialogueでは、どのように改善されていたでしょうか。
2. このケースが難しいのは、なぜだと思いますか。
   bad newに対して患者さんはどのように反応しているでしょうか。

III Comprehension Check

Watch the good dialogue and choose the most appropriate answer to each question on the DVD.

1. **Q:** [   ]
   a. A MacMillan nurse   b. Mr. Rees   c. Mrs. Rees

2. **Q:** [   ]
   a. Panic   b. Fatigue   c. Breast cancer

3. **Q:** [   ]
   a. She feels all right, and doesn't understand it.
   b. She is so shocked that she can't speak.
   c. She's surprised and wants to ask many questions about it.

4. **Q:** [   ]
   a. The nurse asks her to come again next week.
   b. The nurse tells her to go to the desk to make an appointment for the next week.
   c. The nurse tells her not to book an appointment for next week.

IV Complete the Dialogue

Watch the good dialogue again and fill in the blanks.

(N: Nurse P: Patient)

N: Hi, Mrs. Roberts. I'm Isabelle, one of the MacMillan nurses. It's nice to meet you.

P: Oh, yeah, Isabelle, yeah? OK, hello, hi.

N: You (1)_____ last week.

P: Yeah, Mr. Rees.

N: That's right. How did you get on?

P: Well, he was a bit scary. But, he told me a lot of things, but it was so quick, and... it's a lot to remember.

Unit 15   Consultation (Cancer)

N: Did he tell you your (2)_____?

P: Well, he said I had cancer. He said I had breast cancer.

N: That's right. I'm sorry it's been bad news for you.

P: It's (3)_____ _____ _____ a shock.

N: How have you been feeling?

P: I feel OK. I don't understand.

N: Well, often, cancer patients will feel OK. It's natural (4)_____ _____ _____ _____.

P: But I don't know (5)_____ _____ _____ now because I feel OK, and... I'm panicking a bit.

N: There's no need to panic. For the moment, you don't need to do anything. And it's good that you're feeling well in yourself. What I'd like to do is to see you regularly, and hopefully, over (6)_____ _____ _____, we can talk in more detail about what's happening.

P: Because I can ask you about it, then. Things I don't understand, yeah?

N: Of course. You will have (7)_____ _____ as the weeks go by, and we can (8)_____ each of those in turn.

P: OK, yeah, (9)_____ _____ _____.

N: Shall I come and see you next week in your own home?

P: Oh, yeah, yeah, that would be better, I think.

N: So, as you go out to the desk, you can (10)_____ _____ _____, and I'll look forward to seeing you next week.

P: OK, thank you.

V Substitution Practice

Replace the shaded expressions with those below and read them aloud.

1. I don't know what to do.
   - how to use a commode
   - where to go
   - whom to talk to about cancer

2. We'd like to see you regularly.
   - our grandchild very often
   - your family every summer
   - him not so often but regularly

3. We can tackle each question in turn.
   - solve each problem
   - check each smoking area

4. We can talk in more detail about what's happening.
   - your prognosis
   - his kidney cancer
   - his dementia
   - her chronic bronchitis

VI Expand Your Vocabulary

From the box below, choose and write down the English words with the same meaning as the following Japanese words.

肺がん _____ 予後 _____

パニック _____ 診断 _____

喫煙所 _____ 認知症 _____

抱く _____ 腎臓がん _____

家庭内暴力 _____ 慢性気管支炎 _____

```
hold              smoking area         lung cancer
kidney cancer     chronic bronchitis   dementia
prognosis         domestic violence    diagnosis
panic
```

VII Speaking Practice

1. 動画を見て自分で練習してよく覚えましょう。
2. ペアになって役割を交代して練習しましょう。
3. 致命的な病気を知らされた患者さんと看護師のペアになり、どのような質問がされるかを考えて会話を行ってみましょう。

いろいろな表現を覚えましょう

☞ 病名告知後の表現

I'm afraid it's been bad news for you.

I'm afraid you can't really believe the diagnosis.

Please take it easy.

Don't be so nervous, please.

How are you getting on?

How have you been feeling?

How have you been coping?

Often, patients in your situation do feel quite well.

Sometimes, it's quite natural to feel quite well.

You don't need to do anything at the moment.

There are some cancers that can be treated.

We will be able to talk about your cancer in more detail again.

Common Abbreviations

ADL	activities of daily living 日常生活動作
Adm	admission 入院
AIDS	acquired immuno-deficiency syndrome 後天性免疫不全症候群
BM (bm)	bowel movement 便通, 排便
BP	blood pressure 血圧
CC	chief complaint 主訴
CCU	coronary care unit 冠状動脈疾患集中治療病棟(部)
CPR	cardiopulmonary resuscitation 心肺蘇生
CT (CAT)	computerized tomography コンピューター断層撮影
D/C (dc)	discontinue 中止する; discharge 退院
Disc	discharge 退院
ECG (EKG)	electrocardiogram 心電図
F	Fahrenheit 力氏(温度の単位); female 女性
GTT	glucose tolerance test ブドウ糖負荷試験
h (hr)	hour 時間
HR	heart rate 心拍数
ICU	intensive care unit 集中治療部, 集中ケア病棟
I & O	intake and output 摂取量と排泄量
IV	intravenous 静脈内の
lab	laboratory 検査室
M	male 男性
MRI	magnetic resonance imaging 磁気共鳴映像法
OR	operating room 手術室
P (PR)	pulse 脈拍
PE	physical examination 診察, 身体検査
PET	positron-emission tomography ポジトロンCT, 陽電子放出断層撮影
POS	problem-oriented system 問題志向システム
Ps	prescription 処方箋
QOL	quality of life 生活(生命)の質
R (RR)	respiratory rate 呼吸数
RN	registered nurse 登録看護師
ROM	range of motion 可動域
T (temp)	temperature 温度, 体温
TB (TBC)	tuberculosis 結核
TPR	temperature, pulse, respiration 体温, 脈拍, 呼吸
UA	urine test; urinalysis 尿検査
US	ultrasonography 超音波検査

Web動画のご案内 StreamLine

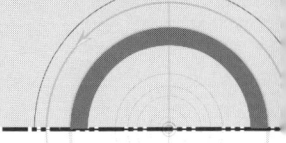

本テキストの映像は、オンラインでのストリーミング再生になります。下記URLよりご利用ください。なお**有効期限は、はじめてログインした時点から1年半**です。

http://st.seibido.co.jp

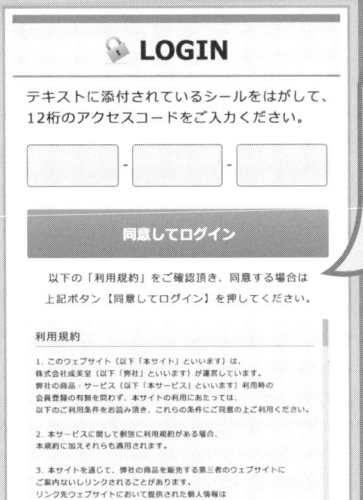

① ログイン画面

テキストに添付されているシールをはがして、12桁のアクセスコードをご入力ください。

巻末に添付されているシールをはがして、アクセスコードをご入力ください。

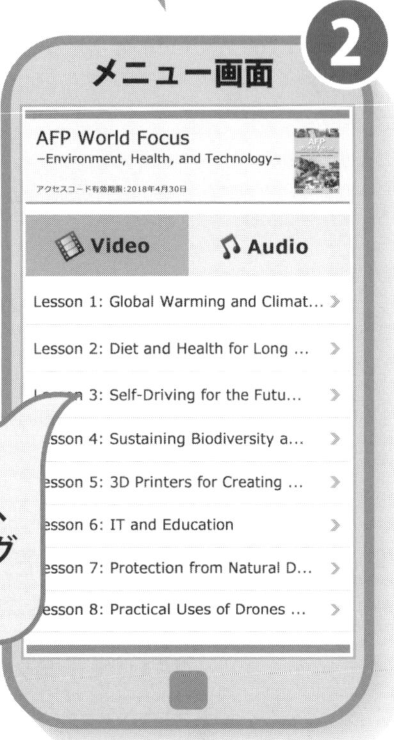

② メニュー画面

AFP World Focus
−Environment, Health, and Technology−
アクセスコード有効期限:2018年4月30日

Video / Audio

Lesson 1: Global Warming and Climat...
Lesson 2: Diet and Health for Long ...
Lesson 3: Self-Driving for the Futu...
Lesson 4: Sustaining Biodiversity a...
Lesson 5: 3D Printers for Creating ...
Lesson 6: IT and Education
Lesson 7: Protection from Natural D...
Lesson 8: Practical Uses of Drones ...

「Video」または「Audio」を選択すると、それぞれストリーミング再生ができます。

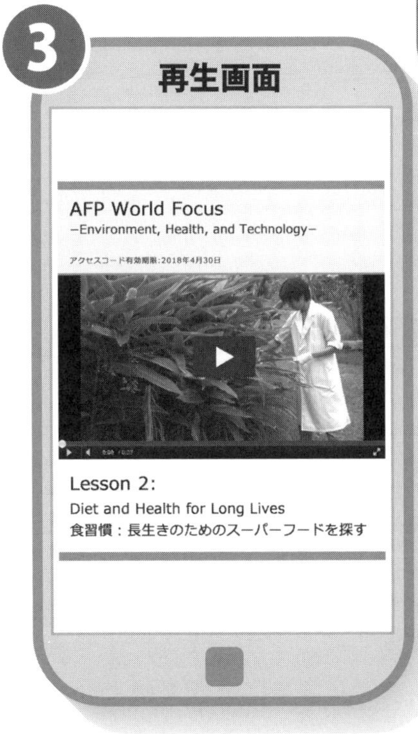

③ 再生画面

AFP World Focus
−Environment, Health, and Technology−
アクセスコード有効期限:2018年4月30日

Lesson 2:
Diet and Health for Long Lives
食習慣：長生きのためのスーパーフードを探す

推奨動作環境

【PC OS】
Windows 7~ / Mac 10.8~

【Mobile OS】
iOS / Android ※Androidの場合は4.x~が推奨

【Desktop ブラウザ】
Internet Explorer 9~ / Firefox / Chrome / Safari / Microsoft Edge

TEXT PRODUCTION STAFF

edited by Kimio Sato	編集 佐藤 公雄
English-language editing by Bill Benfield	英文校閲 ビル・ベンフィールド
cover design by Ruben Frosali	表紙デザイン ルーベン・フロサリ
text design by Ruben Frosali	本文デザイン ルーベン・フロサリ

Everyday English for Nursing on DVD
DVDで学ぶ看護英語

2010年1月20日 初版 発行
2023年3月10日 第15刷 発行

著　者　園城寺 康子　　John Skelton
発行者　佐野 英一郎
発行所　株式会社 成美堂
　　　　〒101-0052　東京都千代田区神田小川町3-22
　　　　TEL 03-3291-2261　FAX 03-3293-5490
　　　　https://www.seibido.co.jp

印刷・製本　倉敷印刷（株）

ISBN 978-4-7919-3120-0　　　　Printed in Japan

・落丁・乱丁本はお取り替えします。
・本書の無断複写は、著作権上の例外を除き著作権侵害となります。

memo

memo

memo

memo